BODYBUILDING SECRETS:

FULL GUIDE TO CREATING A FANTASTIC MALE FIGURE

By

PIERS ERICKSON

Copyright © by PIERS ERICKSON 2023. All rights reserved.

Table Of Contents

Introduction

Building the ideal body involves dedication, hard work, and persistence. As a result, believing in a silver bullet that would transform your body overnight is pointless. The good news is that you may speed up your fitness improvements by following basic workout principles. Whether you want to lose weight, gain muscle mass, or both, these are the workout rules you should follow for the best results.

Health is an important aspect of strength. Everyday activities like getting out of bed, lugging groceries, and pulling a broken-down automobile off the road all demand it. It is described as the capacity to exert the greatest amount of force in the face of a particular, typically external barrier. Developing strength can be beneficial whether you're a younger person looking to lift more weight off the bench or an older senior concerned about standing up from a chair comfortably. Greater strength is associated with reductions in all causes of mortality, according to a recent study. Another study discovered a connection between strength training and better physical function in people with chronic pain.

Controlling body weight and composition is a big problem when it comes to public health and an important obligation for athletes. Technology, the food business, and even the health industry have all gradually pushed individuals toward an unhealthy lifestyle that results in an unfit physique. To compensate, individuals have devised a plethora of strategies for decreasing weight and purportedly being healthy. Some ways are odd, some are unpleasant, and some are plain dangerous. While a healthy lifestyle may necessitate some effort and discipline, it should not be insane, extreme, or miserable. Many people work very hard to maintain a healthy body. Effort is not always the issue. In some circumstances, the issue is that people are entirely misinformed about what constitutes a healthy lifestyle. The purpose of this post is to give a healthy and fun approach to a lean body.

Chapter 1

How to develop a perfect physique.

Working hard, being committed, and being consistent are necessary to develop the ideal physique. Therefore, it is useless to think that there is a magic cure that would make your body alter in an instant. The good news is that you can quicken your fitness improvements by following a few workout recommendations. Here are the training recommendations you should stick to for best results, regardless of whether your goal is to lose weight, gain muscle mass, or both.

Perform light workout

The foundation of each workout is a strong warm-up. A decent warm-up increases body temperature and gets the blood circulating, allowing you to lift greater weight later. Skipping the warm-up is a recipe for disaster because being chilly increases your risk of injury and early weariness. As a result, make sure to warm up properly before your workouts. To properly warm up, begin with light cardio for 5 minutes, such as jogging, biking, or running in place, and then do 5 minutes of simple bodyweight exercises to get your body moving.

Lift Large

The cornerstone of your program should be large compound movements when it comes to the proper lifting techniques. Increases in growth and testosterone hormone levels are brought on by exercises like the deadlift, squat, and bench press, which speed up muscle growth and improve fitness. Additionally, compound motions stimulate a significant number of muscle fibers, increasing the amount of energy expended and the likelihood of fat loss.

Proper Posture

Bad form is one of the main causes of injuries. Bad training form can be disastrous for your training resolution, whether it manifests as fidgeting, an arched back, or any of the other warning signals. As a result, be sure to incorporate proper form habits into your training. Before you start to get huge, get technical. Be open to feedback and ask around for it. Of course, the ideal way to assist you in establishing and maintaining proper form is to hire a personal trainer.

Liberalize your muscles

Utilizing free weights during exercise as opposed to fixed devices results in higher muscle activation and, consequently, better muscle growth. Additionally, free weights are more practical, easier to use, and can help you build strong form habits that can help you avoid injuries and breakthrough performance plateaus. Therefore, use free weights to complete your workouts without much problem rather than wasting time waiting for the Smith machine.

Moment of Tension

The duration of an activity is the main factor affecting muscle growth. Time under tension, or TUT for short, is what that is. Numerous studies have found that the best duration of tension for the greatest amount of muscle growth is between 40 and 60 seconds. If you don't do enough, there won't be any tension. If you exert too much, you run the risk of overtraining your muscles. For best growth, time your sets to fall inside that range.

Frequently Sprint

Long runs have advantages. They support fat-burning and endurance-building. However, they are monotonous and can be time- and muscle-consuming. Fortunately, interval running can make it easier for you to get those advantages.

This style of jogging, which is a form of high-intensity interval training, can help you lose weight, increase metabolism, build lethal lower body strength and speed, and get in the greatest shape of your life. Here's how to continue your interval training runs:

Start by warming up properly.

Run slowly for five minutes while taking deep breaths. Start your first sprint for 45 seconds at 80% of your maximum effort. To recover, jog slowly for an additional 45 seconds. Seven to ten times, repeat the on/off intensity cycle. After the workout, chill down. Jog slowly for five minutes, then stretch.

Accept Change

The same workout program over and over again can only lead to boredom and performance plateaus. Constant change is essential if you want to see success with your training regimen. You must continue to push your body beyond its comfort zone to achieve it. As a result, be careful to advance with each exercise you perform. If you perform 15 reps in one session, raise the load for the following session's 10 or 12 reps. Keep the load the same but reduce the reps to 15, such that each session only involves one variable being altered.

Chapter 2

Easy scientific ways of building strength and muscle.

Strength is an essential component of healthy health. Many daily tasks need it, such as getting out of bed, carrying groceries, or pushing a broken-down car off the road. It is defined as the ability to generate maximum force in the face of a specified and usually external opposition. Knowing how to increase strength might be useful whether you're an older adult concerned about getting out of a chair safely or a younger person attempting a larger bench press.According to a recent study, improved strength is connected with a decrease in all causes of death. Another study found a link between strength training and improved physical function in persons with chronic pain.

Resistance training can be used for a variety of reasons. Others aim to build a better body with larger muscles and perform better in specialized sports. Regardless of your objectives, you may be unsure of the best way to improve your strength. It is vital to recognize that long-term consistency is required to achieve results and that key variables must be controlled in order to challenge your body to lift heavier loads. Increasing the weight, shifting the number of repetitions each set, adjusting the number of days you lift, changing how long you rest between sets, and adjusting the number of sets you perform are some of the reasons. The themes are addressed in the following manner to develop strength.

How long does it take to gain muscle mass?

Long-term consistency is essential when it comes to gaining strength. According to a recent study, it usually takes between six and fifteen weeks to observe any noticeable strength gains. Nonetheless, because your brain adapts to exercise, you may experience strength gains in the first few weeks of training. These instant strength gains are more common in untrained people than in skilled people.

It's important to understand the distinction between muscle and strength building. The purpose of muscle building is to increase muscular size, commonly known as causing muscle hypertrophy. This is not always the purpose of strength training. Appreciable muscular hypertrophy typically takes at least eight to sixteen weeks, depending on nutrition, intensity, frequency, and other factors such as age and gender.

Strength

Strength training's primary purpose is to teach your body to adapt to lifting bigger loads. You can run a test to see if your strength has improved. You can, for example, see if your 1RM lift of a given exercise, such as the bench press or squat, improves with time. In other words, as you advance, you may determine if you can execute one repetition of an exercise with increasing loads. According to research, improving strength demands lifting loads that are more than or equal to 60% of your 1RM load. If you have previous training experience, loads of at least 80% of your 1RM load may create superior strength increases.

Current suggestions for improving strength using resistance training are to perform 1-8 repetitions until muscular failure (inability to perform another repetition). According to research, you should do 3-6 of these sets every workout. According to one study, three-minute rest periods are ideal for creating strength changes. However, resting for 1-3 minutes between sets may be more useful in terms of time savings.

Keep in mind that strength training will differ depending on the individual. It is affected by previous training history, injuries, age, motivation, and other factors. As a result, it's necessary to tailor your training parameters to your abilities, time constraints, and motivation level. If you're over 45, for example, you might benefit from lesser loads, such as 60% of your 1-RM load.

Hypertrophy

The purpose of hypertrophy training, as previously stated, is to increase muscular size. Maximum lifting may not be required as part of this regimen. One study, for example, discovered that hypertrophy can occur with loads as little as 30% of 1RM. Nonetheless, higher loads resulted in greater muscle size growth. The key aspect is maintained training at a high level till muscular failure.

According to a 2016 study, muscle mass rose when a participant performed three sets of eight to twelve repetitions to muscular failure. If your goal is to build muscle, you should rest for 1-3 minutes between sets, just as you would while trying to enhance strength. Interestingly, some research claims that resting longer between sets improves muscle endurance.

Muscular stamina

The ability to move a submaximal load while avoiding muscle fatigue is referred to as muscular endurance. Loads that are 40-60% of your 1RM are commonly used in training to develop muscle endurance. This increases the physiologic efficiency of the muscle, allowing it to conduct repeated contractions without becoming exhausted. This helps you to push your body for extended periods, such as when jogging or swimming. Muscular endurance training often consists of executing 2-3 sets of 15 or more repetitions. Rest intervals are typically shorter, lasting 30-60 seconds.

Power

Muscle power is the ability to move yourself or an object with force and quickness. Sprinting, discus throwing, slam-ball workouts, and jumping are just a few examples. The appropriate training loads vary based on the exercise. Power movements like the squat, for example, and explosive lifts like the power clean respond well to weights of 30-70% of your 1RM. Meanwhile, explosive sports like jumping benefit from smaller loads that are roughly 30% of your 1RM.

Power training repetitions are designed to improve strength and speed, and you should avoid training to muscle failure. This sort of training usually consists of 1-3 sets of 4-10 reps. The rest times are longer, lasting 3 minutes or more, allowing you to fully recuperate before continuing. In contrast training, it can be combined with strong resistance sets. This can aid in muscle development and pre-fatigue. Using a larger resistance set in conjunction with a much lighter speed-based movement improves performance.

How to maintain your strength objectives with nutrition.

If you want to increase your strength and muscle mass, you need to increase your protein consumption. According to recent studies, increasing muscle mass and strength can be aided by consuming up to 0.73 grams of protein per pound (1.6 grams per kilogram) of body weight per day. Any more than this will be eliminated in your urine and will provide no additional benefits. A 155-pound (70-kg) person, for example, can benefit from up to 112 grams of protein per day. Lean meat, chicken, and fish, as well as legumes, dairy, and grains, can provide this. You can also take protein supplements, which are often made from soy, pea, or whey protein.

It may be beneficial to change your protein sources to improve your body's intake. This will offer diversity to your diet and ensure that you get all of the different amino acids, often known as the protein building blocks. The above advice does necessitate a sufficient workout stimulus to justify the increased intake. In other words, eating this much protein without also working out at a high enough intensity is unlikely to trigger more muscle building. Those who exercise less vigorously may not require more than 0.36 grams per pound (0.8 grams per kilogram) of body weight per day.

In addition to acquiring enough protein, you should strive for a well-balanced diet. This includes whole grains and other high-quality carbohydrates, as well as fruits and vegetables that give fiber, vitamins, and minerals. A balanced diet can boost your health and help avoid disease in addition to powering your exercises.

Chapter 3

The scientific ways of getting lean.

When it comes to the general public's health and the health of athletes, controlling body weight and body composition is a major concern. People's adoption of an unhealthy lifestyle that results in an unfit physique has been gradually encouraged by technology, the food business, and even the health industry itself. People have developed numerous techniques for reportedly being healthy and decreasing weight to make up for this. Some techniques are strange, uncomfortable, and even unhealthy. A healthy lifestyle should not be outrageous, extreme, insane, or unhappy, however, it does need some effort and discipline. Many people make great efforts to maintain physical health. Often, effort is not the problem. In some circumstances, the issue is that people have erroneous ideas about what constitutes a healthy lifestyle. This essay aims to outline a route to a slender body that is both fun and healthful.

First is weight control.

The image is straightforward all around. the difference between the calories burnt and those consumed. When you burn more calories than you take in, you lose weight. People are generally aware of this. You can easily manage your calorie intake. Although it might not seem straightforward, it is. Lower calorie intake results from eating less food. Numerous dietary tactics can assist in limiting caloric intake, but we'll pass over those since this essay isn't actually about learning how to eat less.

People frequently believe it is easy to regulate the body's calorie expenditure. More exercise results in more caloric expenditure. Isn't that all there is to it? One of the main worries is this. Many individuals think that the only thing that influences how many calories they burn is exercise. It appears like the only method to reduce weight is to eat little and exercise a lot. As a result, millions of individuals exercise excessively and starve themselves to maintain a healthy weight. This image is seriously flawed in some way. Because it is partially controlled by your body, which is quite complex, the calories outside of the equation are not all that simple.Certain fundamental principles must be understood. First off, your body constantly expels calorics. Always. Every second from the moment of creation in your mother's womb until the moment you take your last breath, your body burns calories to maintain life and carry out each cell's specific role.

The second is that your body controls its metabolism.

It can alter how quickly it uses energy. It does not calculate how many calories it should burn using a BMR calculator. It responds to stimuli and acts on impulses for survival. Exercise can make the body burn calories, but it's only one of several factors. Similar to how you cannot consciously control your heart rate, you cannot consciously control your metabolism. It's critical to realize that your body can operate at a variety of metabolic rates. We don't fully comprehend all of the mechanisms that regulate metabolism.

False beliefs

We can debunk some of the incorrect assumptions about weight control as we go over these facts. For instance, it is absurd to eat and then require activity to burn off the calories. The body continuously expels calories. Energy can be used without exercise. You will die if you work out enough to expend every calorie you consume. not metaphorically. Literally. You'll stop having a life. People worry far too much about how many calories they burn when exercising. Say you love working out and spend two hours working out every day. There are 22 hours left. Which influences metabolism more? 22 or 2 hours? The amount of calories burned while exercising is negligible. The rate at which the body burns calories throughout the other 90% of the day is significantly more significant. I figure that on days when I work out, no more than 20% of my energy is used up by physical exercise.

Diet

It is not advisable to force oneself to go without food all the time. The body will gradually lower its metabolism to match your intake. Because of this, drastically reducing calories only leads to short-term weight loss rather than the long-term lean body most individuals desire. To survive on insufficient calories, the body slows down its metabolic rate when it feels hungry. This reaction includes an increased propensity to retain fat and burn muscle for energy. This does not imply that undereating will result in weight gain. Let's be clear: Eating very little will cause you to lose weight. It indicates that losing weight through fasting results in a body that is less slim and muscular than losing weight through methods that encourage a quick metabolism and the preservation of muscle mass. In other words, when people starve themselves to lose weight, they often end up thin but not lean because they burn off muscle instead of fat, and they also cut down their energy consumption.

As a result, individuals have a higher chance of gaining weight quickly and in the form of fat rather than muscle. Additionally, a decreased metabolic rate is undesirable since it indicates that the body is exerting less effort to maintain the health and functionality of its structures and organs. Want wounds? Want to be ill? Do you want to feel awful? Give up eating. Eating as little as you can stand while engaging in as much cardio as you can is a common weight loss strategy. This method results in bodies that aren't particularly lean, aren't particularly slender, don't look nice, don't feel good, and are outright unhealthy.

What are the healthiest ways to maintain a fit weight and a lean body, then? We must complete two key tasks.

1. Having a quick metabolism should be the aim rather than aiming to ingest extremely few calories. Because it enables you to eat, this has several benefits. It gives you a lot of leeway when it comes to establishing a calorie deficit to shed fat or weight. You can consume a lot of food and yet lose weight if you have a rapid metabolism. Even eating certain unhealthy foods won't stop you from losing weight. It gives a lot of latitude for dietary choices. This significantly improves life quality and reduces stress. Not that you shouldn't pay attention to what you eat at all, but which is simpler to maintain? A diet of 1,500 calories or 2,500 calories? A rapid metabolism makes it much simpler to attain and keep a trim figure. Additionally, it is healthy. It shows that the body is actively repairing itself. Energy is needed for a variety of functions, including muscle repair, ligament and tendon strengthening, bone hardening, organ tissue regeneration, and disease prevention. If the body has enough energy from meals to use rather than constantly being in survival mode, it can accomplish these activities more quickly and fully. Greater health and a much better chance of having a low body fat percentage are made possible by eating a lot and exercising a lot. It is a vital necessity in gencral for athletes. The physical demands of playing, practicing, and training for a sport are great. You'd best hope that as a result of the stress, your body is working hard to maintain itself. Otherwise, you are depleting your body without regenerating it. That will only lead to disaster and subpar sports performance.

2. We also need to sway the body to prioritize muscle growth over fat storage. This has clear advantages for both physical performance and attractiveness. How can we accomplish these two goals? I won't even try to discuss all the factors that affect metabolism, fat storage, and muscle growth because the human body is an incredibly complicated entity. I just want to offer some general tips on nutrition and fitness.

EXERCISE

Higher intensity and extensive muscular activity are the qualities of exercise that produce the best results. These two elements cause a stronger physiological reaction. The term "intensity" describes the amount of effort and muscle tension involved along with the level of effort. Because it requires the most physical effort to produce the most muscular tension, heavy strength training is the most intense physical activity. Heavy, large-scale strength training exercises like squats and deadlifts are the best stimulants of metabolism. Olympic lifting, med ball tosses, jumps, sprints, and playing sports with a lot of effort are more instances of rigorous full-body training. Anything that uses its maximum amount of force is intense. This exercise takes the most recuperation time since it places the most physical and physiological strain on the body. A lot of energy is expended during the recuperation phase. The most muscular growth is stimulated by high-intensity exercise. Even when it is not being used, muscle mass significantly contributes to metabolic rate. (Men typically find it easier to become and maintain a lean body because of this.) Therefore, high-intensity exercise increases metabolism AND tilts the body toward maintaining and gaining muscle. Conveniently, people are appealing because of the same musculature. Both men and women may agree on that. Ladies, starving yourself and riding the stationary bike won't give you great legs and butt. Instead, spend time getting comfortable with the track and the barbell. To top it all off, you may reap the rewards of high-intensity training without having to put in a lot of time at the gym. For both men and women, a solid three hours per week of full-body strength exercise may do wonders for metabolic rate and the growth of aesthetically pleasing musculature.

Unfortunately, cardio, or low-intensity exercise, has long been the most widely used method for losing weight. According to science, this is supported by the fact that low-intensity exercise uses fat to supply a greater proportion of the required energy. People engage in fat-burning activity because they desire to lose weight. This kind of thinking is flawed because, once again, we do not have complete control over our bodies. Protein and carbohydrates can both be stored as fat by the body. It makes no difference how much fat is burned during a workout because any of the macronutrients can be stored as fat. The body is trained to be efficient by long-term, low-intensity exercise, which includes storing an effective fuel source. Efficiency is very important in a food-limited survival circumstance. Efficiency, however, is detrimental while striving to build a lean body. Efficiency means that the body doesn't gain muscular mass while burning fewer calories. On the other hand, high-intensity exercise teaches the body how to use and store carbs, a useful food source. The term proficiency refers to the body using a lot of energy to do a task exceptionally well. excellent work. using a great deal of energy. Looks good, doesn't it? The best sort of exercise for boosting metabolism and reducing fat storage is high-intensity exercise, which is also the best for sculpting a lean physique. The body will be more slim if it is largely acclimated to high-intensity exercise, but this does not imply that all cardio is undesirable. Here are a few studies that back up that assertion: Even with rigorous caloric restriction, periodized resistance training enhances the quality of weight reduction.

Several extremely popular activities are just not intense enough for those looking to get healthy. Let's be clear first. In particular, for general health, any exercise is preferable to none. But not all activity is created equal when it comes to getting a lean physique. The elliptical machine is conceivably the worst of them. The elliptical machine is the physical embodiment of every misconception about weight loss. People may "work out" comfortably for an hour without stopping because it is so simple. I thought the secret to losing weight was to exercise for a very long time. likewise starving yourself, correct? Wrong! Exercise on an elliptical machine is about as time-wasting as it gets. No matter how hard you try, nothing will change. The device moves on its own. An elliptical has no capacity for intensity. Those devices are awful. They should all be sunk to the bottom of the ocean, in my opinion, although it would probably result in fish that were out of shape. So I'll just declare that they ought to all be destroyed. Relocating on. Biking. The rider decides how intense to be. It is more advantageous to bike faster or to increase the resistance on a stationary bike. The elliptical is less effective than sitting there for an hour cycling your legs against air resistance. Walking. Not enough intensity, but speed is preferred. Running. The runner decides how hard to go. It is more intense and advantageous to run vigorously for 15 minutes than to plod along for an hour. Are athletes who run in condition typically? Yes, the hard-running competitors. Female cross-country runners run 5Ks under 6:00 miles per hour, even at the high school level. That exercise is challenging. There is no doubt that it is intense enough. However, the "runners" you see plodding down the sidewalk at 4 mph usually aren't in fantastic shape. I just want to be clear once more. No exercise is harmful to your health or attempts to lose weight, I'm not claiming that. But I'm suggesting that a lot of the activity individuals perform isn't the best for getting a slim physique. Muscle growth and maintenance should be the primary goals of exercise, not fat or calorie burning.

NUTRITION

Exercise and diet both need to be addressed to achieve a lean physique. Being athletic and attractive as well as having a rapid metabolism depends on building and retaining muscular mass. We've known for a long time that consuming more calories generally enables the body to grow more tissue. However, since protein is a component of muscle, a high-protein diet promotes the body to create muscle rather than store fat. A high-protein diet makes the body more inclined to grow muscle. Even better, recent studies have demonstrated that a high-protein diet paired with resistance training enables the maintenance of muscle mass even when there is a caloric deficit. In the subsequent study, the subjects who consumed twice as much protein under a calorie deficit grew muscle mass while losing more fat mass. When paired with vigorous exercise and a calorie deficit, higher dietary protein promotes greater lean mass increase and fat mass loss.

We require how much protein?

According to the research, it appears that exceeding 2.2 grams per kilogram or 1 gram every pound of body weight is beneficial for weight/fat loss. To build a slim body, meeting this need comes first in terms of diet. Remember that the need for protein rises with more frequent, more severe activity. We want to keep our metabolic rate high while simultaneously preserving our muscular mass. If it does not provide a lot of energy, the body will not burn a lot of energy. You can't eat 2,000 calories a day and continue to burn 4,000. The body won't make that happen. It contradicts survival instincts. Simply consuming a lot of food is the next important dietary rule to follow. Contrary to popular belief, a high metabolic rate requires a lot of food consumption. A highly active athlete may be able to maintain weight with a daily caloric intake of their body weight in pounds multiplied by 20 as a rough approximation.

Avoid starving yourself, Don't miss any meals.

You shouldn't base your decision to eat or not on your appetite. No snack should be considered a meal. Don't base your food selection on what contains the fewest calories. Calories aren't all terrible. The body demands food. In a nutshell. You must eat. This will lead to a quick metabolic rate when combined with a suitable exercise regimen. This will explain why your eating habits won't always be great. A quick metabolism can make up for a little pizza, cookie, etc. On the other hand, there is no chance if you turn your body into an efficient machine. Too many people have the misconception that calories are harmful. They view any means of avoiding them as advantageous. It's a success if they can go from supper to bed without eating. Even better if they can skip breakfast. They view everything containing fat as being "bad for you." They consistently select the diet or light choice. Any departure from the low-calorie plan must be made up for with exercise. To force their body to burn fat, they starve themselves, but their bodies merely end up being more and more efficient. It becomes better at avoiding calorie burning. It strives to cling onto fat for survival, burns muscle for energy, and desires junk food because it is so low on calories. This is a useless strategy for getting a slender body. The more radical it becomes, the less likely it is to succeed, and the sicker the body becomes. Yet another time. You must eat.

Therefore, if you want to lose weight, you must reduce your caloric intake to make up the difference. The greatest strategy to sustain and maintain weight loss, however, is to first develop a rapid metabolic rate by eating a lot and engaging in high-intensity activity. This is due to metabolic adaptations to calorie restriction. So, when attempting to lose weight, go slowly. That entails eating enough protein to retain muscle mass while maintaining a slight caloric deficit as opposed to starving yourself. It could also entail a sporadic approach to weight loss.

Let's have a quick discussion on what to eat.

In a perfect world, we would only consume plant-based meals, animal products, and natural sources of fats (such as meat, eggs, and nuts). Sadly, our world is not one in which we can spend all day choosing wonderful food from plants and hunting for wild animals. Even our "natural" meals are frequently altered by the food business. Therefore, it is likely that your diet will not be flawless. Just try your best to obtain as much of your nourishment from natural sources as you can. If you must eat less than optimally to satisfy your protein and calorie requirements, so be it. However, I do advise staying away from alcoholic beverages, fried foods, and sugary desserts. I won't address the numerous purported terrible issues with meat, dairy, gluten, genetically modified foods, etc.

We must therefore adhere to four nutritional principles.

Each day, consume 1 gram of protein per pound of body weight.

Consume a lot of calories (for athletes, this may be BW x 20).

Eat a lot of plant-based foods and sources of protein.

Stay away from junk food.
A person who adheres to these guidelines and regularly engages in vigorous exercise will eventually achieve good general health and a rapid metabolic rate. If you want to lose weight, go by these recommendations but cut back on your caloric intake. If you want to gain weight, eat more. In either case, adhering to these rules is the best method to achieve leanness and health.

For athletes who need to reduce their weight or body fat, here are a few tips:

First off, the exercise component of the equation is already taken care of if you participate in and train for your sport. The answer isn't to exercise more. You should focus your energy on improving your diet. Second, the immediate impact weight loss will have on athleticism is difficult to anticipate. Long-term benefits of becoming lean include improved health and athleticism brought on by the bulk in your body. That is not what extra fat does. You only feel heavier as a result. However, losing weight can result in a loss of strength or simply a poor response to exercise. Depending on the circumstance, changes in body weight and strength may or may not immediately result in improved athletic performance. A high-protein diet is essential to maximize the benefits of weight loss for athleticism since it helps preserve muscle mass.

Nature's Life

What I'm advocating ought to be simple. Exercise is a natural, start. Humans were created to move. Exercise provides a broad number of health benefits because the body was made to move, not because it's some amazing technique someone developed. The issue is that people do not need to travel very much in today's world. It promotes indolence. The majority of individuals spend their days inactive. Children must sit in class all day, complete their assignments, read, and study. They are finally qualified to spend the entire day at work once they reach adulthood and complete their education. Most people don't have much time to devote to exercise, so you need to make that little bit of time productive. High-intensity exercise is crucial for this reason. An hour of aerobics cannot make up for a whole day of inactivity. Nowhere near. On the other hand, your body can endure a lot of physical stress from 60 minutes of strength exercise. Second, natural nourishment is all that constitutes proper nutrition. When you are hungry, eat. eat food that is provided by the earth. It's incredibly easy. You'll have a healthy body if you lead a natural life. There aren't any strange techniques or "insane fat-burning secrets" here, as you'll see. Furthermore, this is hardly a rigorous willpower test. The way of life I suggest is pretty delightful. You don't need to skip meals, spend hours working out every day, consume only special food that is sent to you by mail, cut down carbs or fat, take pills to burn fat, sprinkle magic powder on each plate, or track your food points. Instead, you get up and spend the entire day eating things that make your body feel wonderful. The body of a person aspires to health. We don't need to devise bizarre strategies to get it to behave in this way. Simply lead a natural existence.

Chapter 4

Requirements for effective nutrition.

Meal planning is a crucial part of nutrition regimens and has grown in popularity among those who want to reduce weight and pursue other fitness objectives. Nutrition can be very confusing because there are so many different alternatives for personalized meal plans or diet regimens. It's not entirely accurate to assume that 20% of activity and 80% of food create benefits. For the best outcomes, both food and exercise require complete commitment. Let's take a closer look at how to create a diet plan that works with each client's lifestyle and exercise routine.

Throughout this essay, keep your personal trainer's scope of practice in mind. What you are permitted to provide clients in your capacity as a trainer is subject to rules and regulations that differ between states and even gyms. Refer out if you're uncertain.

Elements of a Meal Plan

Although they can differ, the words "nutrition plan" and "meal plan" are frequently used interchangeably. Meal plans frequently involve more numbers and expose consumers to greater health hazards. This method of meal planning may promote unhealthy eating patterns that result in eating disorders. A client's body may eventually stop responding to hunger and fullness cues. This results from worrying excessively about macronutrient targets and meal timing. A customer is more likely to disregard their body's normal signals when they adhere to a strict eating plan for a period. The food plan starts to take precedence over what the body wants and needs. It will be challenging for clients to maintain precise calorie and macronutrient quantities when following a diet plan like this. These circumstances occur when clients eat all of their daily caloric allowances before lunchtime and then decide to skip meals for the remainder of the day.

Depending on the sort of client, their objectives, and their circumstances, counting macronutrients while adhering to a meal plan may be advantageous. Although it is just one part of meal planning, it differs from comprehensive nutrition plans or how-to manuals. Instead of only considering how much food a client should consume, nutrition programs also consider the quality of the foods they choose. For a client to experience long-term weight loss and outcomes, how they feel is more crucial. You can modify a client's diet based on the indications of hunger and fullness they experience, as well as any digestive issues. The scope of calorie monitoring makes it impossible to pinpoint the specific foods that are causing digestive problems.

Clients can achieve optimum health within their bodies with the aid of diet regimens that emphasize the quality of food rather than just reaching macronutrient targets.

They can identify foods that boost energy, promote satisfaction, and sharpen the mind. A client can decide when to eat and when not to eat depending on their body's natural clock when they have a tailored meal plan that offers this.

The benefit of developing a nutrition strategy

Nutritional programs give clients flexibility and control over their diets, which boosts their confidence. Clients will feel less stress and worry if they are more secure about their nutrition.

Skip the calorie-counting

Without having to keep track of everything a customer consumes, nutrition regimens create results. A client should take a well-balanced diet into account when selecting meals to eat. Eating balanced meals is simple when you eat a diet rich in fruits, vegetables, lean proteins, whole grains, and other micronutrient-dense foods.

Meal preparation

Giving clients the option of what to eat and how to schedule their meals is possible with a guided diet plan. Your client won't have to eat the same thing repeatedly thanks to the huge variety of meal options. A busy client's ability to stay organized and dedicated to their diet plan might be improved with meal planning. Although not suitable for everyone, this style of planning and preparation can make clients' diet regimens simpler to adhere to.

Glucose Levels

Eating habits and diet directly affect this. Affecting underlying anxiety and stress levels are sudden variations in blood sugar levels. Blood sugar levels might rise or fall depending on the food a client chooses to eat and when they eat it. Carbohydrates are one group of foods that directly affect health. By eating frequent little meals or snacks and refraining from missing meals, clients can maintain stable blood sugar levels. Dietary sugary meals raise insulin levels. Limit your intake of complex carbohydrates, and choose healthy foods like fruits and vegetables. Antioxidants and omega-3 fatty acids are nutrients that help the body control stress and inflammation.

Formulating a Nutrition Plan

You must first gather information about your family history, food allergies, medications, dietary supplements, occupation, nutritional preferences, and current eating patterns before you can create a diet plan. By taking these factors into account, you can avoid putting restrictions on a client's diet. Clients' sleeping hours, mealtimes, and food choices are all crucial factors.

A client will eat more phytonutrients, vitamins, and minerals if their food and diet options are more varied. Vegetable sources are a major source of several of these nutrients.

All customers, regardless of age, should have access to nutrition programs, and you should work to dispel any fallacies and fad diets that our clients may have. This will enable them to adopt the new strategy we suggest without hesitation. A balanced diet that includes lean meats, fruits, vegetables, whole grains, complex carbs, and healthy fats can be beneficial for every client. Your customers will consume micronutrients if they follow a well-balanced diet. When planning meals, make sure to keep an eye on your intake of salt, sugar, alcohol, and trans or saturated fats.

Include a food list that categorizes foods in a client's diet plan. A well-balanced meal is made up of these components. Instead of only offering serving-size suggestions, accompany this with comparison tables for portions. Customers may prepare meals more quickly and effectively without having to worry about measuring or weighing their ingredients thanks to this.

Choose one lean meat from the options and consume a portion the size of your fist.

Choose any lean meat and consume 6 ounces of cooked meat.

Utilizing Support Systems Can Help You Achieve Nutritional Success.

Children may be a significant factor in a client's diet plan and food journal. Making entertaining and wholesome snacks for kids might help clients establish a support system. Allow kids to choose whatever fruits and veggies they wish to include in each meal and set objectives for them to eat the rainbow every day. Plan each meal to assist you to avoid making poor food decisions at the last minute. The partners must also be on board. They can be a big help in preventing harmful items from being brought into the house. It's important to select baked or grilled cooking methods. Another important component of nutrition planning is replacing sugary drinks like soda or juice with flavored sparkling water and sweets like ice cream sundaes with yogurt parfaits.

Additionally, as a trainer, it is our responsibility to identify eating patterns and foods that sneak calories into our clients' diets. You can identify these eating tendencies by food logging and take appropriate action. Because they don't feel in control of their meal plan when they feel forced to log everything they eat, they continuously worry about it. They can develop nutrition independence if they keep track of the food they eat and correlate it with how it makes them feel.

Resources and Tools for Formulating a Nutrition Plan

There are no longer any justifications for clients and trainers not to be organized, given how quickly technology is developing. The emotional stress that a meal plan can put on clients can be reduced with the use of apps. You may make nutrition plans that are practical and simple to follow with these and numerous more meal-planning apps. Some apps enable your client to put up a website according to the dict you suggest. They take into account their desire for a certain number of meals throughout the day, food preferences, food allergies, and weight loss goals.

Others can create grocery lists based on a meal your client selects, making it simpler for the client to go grocery shopping. They may even offer the cooking instructions for each meal. They can be used to make meals that you can enter into the app. This enables you to become adaptable and change your diet and lifestyle to fit theirs.

Don't be reluctant, as a trainer, to ask medical experts for help creating a nutrition plan. Nutritionists and registered dietitians can support you in improving your meal preparation. Your professional credibility is not diminished by this. It demonstrates to your consumers how professionally you conduct yourself and how much you care about their weight loss and outcomes. Become an ISSA Nutritionist to master the science of nutrition. This certification enables you to advance your nutritional knowledge and supports all career options in the fitness industry. You will learn about actual nutritional situations that clients frequently encounter. It offers you the authority to switch between a client's program's fitness and dietary goals.

Chapter 5

Practices that help transform your physique quickly.

You can live a better life and get fit by changing your body. All it takes to improve your health and appearance is to make small changes to your everyday workout and eating routines. You must first determine your basal metabolic rate (BMR) to determine how many calories you must consume or expend daily. When you begin your routines, make sure you have an attainable objective in mind so that you are prepared for success. Your physique will appear tidy and you'll feel stronger once you're done!

Among the techniques is setting goals.
1. Establish a clear and realistic aim for what you want to achieve. It is essential to identify the ultimate result of your fitness regimen when you first begin to consider changing the way your body looks. Decide if you want to acquire a certain proportion of muscle or reduce a certain amount of weight. You'll be more likely to stay with your objective if you write it down. For instance, you might want to increase your muscle mass by 5% or shed 10 lb (4.5 kg). Discuss your weight loss objectives with your doctor to see if they have any questions or remarks. Different body types and training regimens are needed for various goals, such as powerlifting or

marathon running. Make sure your smaller objectives contribute to your overall goal.

2. Set a realistic timetable for yourself to accomplish your objectives. Set small and long-term goals for yourself because changing your body can take some time to complete. You can often burn 1-2 lb (0.45-0.91 kg) of fat or add 14-12 lb (0.11-0.23 kg) of muscle every week if you work hard. Determine your timetable based on the number of pounds you can burn off each week. You can set your target between 5 and 10 weeks if, for instance, you wish to lose 10 lb (4.5 kg). If you intend to add 3 lb (1.4 kg) of muscle, give yourself 6–12 weeks to do it. When you first begin training, gaining muscle mass is simpler, but it gets harder over time. Your body type and age may have an impact on how quickly your muscles grow during exercise. Younger people have a faster rate of muscular growth than people in their 40s or 50s.

3. To keep track of your meals and calorie consumption, keep a food journal. For the week, record every meal you consume. Include any food or beverages you may have. When the week is over, check how many calories you consumed so you can determine your average daily intake. Pay attention to specific portion quantities to determine where you are overeating. You can track your daily intake and nutrition using a variety of applications.

4. Make yourself accountable for your goals by using a fitness app. You may track your objectives and get reminders to help you reach them using a variety of phone apps. Install a couple of applications and try to enter your desired weight loss. Utilize the app to keep track of your nutrition, record your workouts, and determine your progress toward your goal.

You may test out MyFitnessPal, Fitbit, and Lose It! for free.

5. Determine your BMR to determine how many calories you require daily. Your body consumes calories on its own to function or at your basal metabolic rate, or BMR. To calculate your BMR, measure your height in inches and weight in pounds. Then, utilize an internet calculator. You must eat fewer calories than your BMR if you want to lose weight, but slightly more calories than your BMR if you want to grow muscle.

Using an internet calculator, you may figure out your BMR. Your level of activity during the day has an impact on your BMR as well. Because they only consider your height and weight and ignore your bone structure, BMR measurements can be unreliable.

Making an effort to lose weight

1. To lose weight, consume 500 fewer calories per day than your BMR. Eating fewer calories than you burn each day is the only way to reduce weight and burn fat. To assist in regulating your caloric intake and help you control your appetite, try intermittent fasting rather than eating three substantial meals throughout the day. Choose a 12- to 16-hour window each day during which you abstain from eating, such as the interval between 8 p.m. and 8 a.m. the following day. If your BMR is 2,000 calories, for instance, you should try to consume roughly 1,500 calories daily.

Use a calorie-counting app to help you plan your daily meals.
Consume only the portions specified on the food's packaging to prevent overeating.

2. Pick foods that are high in protein and unsaturated fat. Include foods like tofu, beans, chicken, eggs, fish, and other lean protein sources in your diet. Keep butter and other saturated fats out of your diet. Instead, substitute almonds, avocado, and olive oil in your meals to help keep them healthy. Vegetable oil butter is an option if you prefer eating butter. Fast food and processed snacks should be avoided because they may include hidden sugars and fats. To determine whether the items you purchase are healthy for you, check the nutrition labels on each one.

Use apps for weight loss or the internet to find lean recipes.

3. Lessen your intake of simple carbohydrates. White bread, white rice, and baked products like cookies are examples of simple carbohydrates. Simple sugars included in simple carbohydrates, which are easier for the body to digest, might cause weight gain. To help your body gradually feel less hungry, try whole grain bread, brown rice, oatmeal, or quinoa with your meal. Fruit and vegetables are excellent providers of complex carbohydrates.

4. Reduce sugar intake. It's best to limit your intake of sweets as much as you can if you're trying to lose weight because the sugar they contain can eventually transform into fat. Try eating a slice of fruit if you're craving sugar instead. Once you eliminate sugar from your diet, you'll start to experience improvements right away.[9] Stay away from sugary beverages like soda and fruit juices and switch to water in their place.

5. Select fresh produce and fruit.
Natural sugars and complex carbohydrates found in fruits and vegetables make them a nutritious substitute for sweets. Eat some fruit with your breakfast, such as an apple or banana, to get your day started. Consider adding additional healthy veggies to the rest of your meals, like spinach, cauliflower, and Brussels sprouts. Fruit juices shouldn't be consumed because they are sweet and lack the nutrients of a piece of fruit. To avoid purchasing unhealthy snacks, bring some fruit with you. Avoid bringing cash with

you to use on vending machine snacks if you are easily tempted by them.

6. Constantly sip on water. To keep your body operating properly and to flush away extra salt, stay hydrated throughout the day. If you're dehydrated, you'll feel more energized and, if you're seeking anything, less hungry. To keep your body healthy, make sure to drink water every day. Drink water throughout and after a vigorous workout when you are perspiring.

7. Begin lifting weights at least three times each week. Lean muscle burns more calories while you're resting, even if lifting weights increases muscle mass and could make you overweight. To build and tone your muscles safely, start with smaller weights and a high rep range to strengthen your connective tissues. Every other day,

weight training with a different muscle area in mind. Try raising the weight or performing more reps for each set as you get used to your current rep range or weight. Instead of doing your workouts on consecutive days, space them out throughout the week. Give yourself at least a day in between each weight training session.

8. Perform cardio exercises 5–6 times per week. Cardio exercises aid in calorie burning and heart health. Include activities like swimming, jumping rope, and running. Aim to perform a 30- to 45-minute cardio workout most days of the week to burn fat. Plan one leisure day each week so that your body has time to unwind.

Use cardio as a quick warm-up before a strenuous exercise session, such as a 10-minute jog before a set of weightlifting.

9. Interval training exercises can help you burn calories quickly. By alternating between high-intensity bursts and recuperation intervals, high-intensity interval training boosts your body's ability to burn calories. After warming up, you might, for instance, sprint for 1 minute, stroll for 2 minutes, and repeat for a 20-minute workout. Your body can continue to burn fat for the following 24 hours with the support of this kind of training. Before beginning interval training, make sure your body is warmed up to avoid stressing or harming your muscles. After your workout, cool down to gradually lower your heart rate.

Muscle growth and toning.

1. To gain muscle, consume up to 500 more calories each day than your BMR. Your exercises won't help you increase muscle mass if you don't consume an excess of up to 500 calories per day for muscle growth. Eat only a modest amount more than you need to avoid gaining body fat. Use a meal journal or a phone app to keep track of how many calories you consume. Aim to eat fewer calories to reduce weight before trying to gain muscle if you're overweight. To determine how many calories you must consume to achieve your goals, you may choose to gradually increase your intake. You'll get fat if you eat too many extra calories.

2. Consume 0.8 grams of protein every pound (0.45 kilograms) of body weight. Since it aids in the development of lean muscles, protein is crucial to your diet. You can help yourself fulfill your daily protein goal by eating things like chicken, fish, yogurt, and beans. To reap the most advantages, consume the protein as soon as possible after working out. If you weigh 150 lb (68 kg), for instance, you should eat 120 g of protein per day.

3. Opt for complex carbohydrates over simple ones. White bread and other simple carbohydrates are simple for your body to break down, therefore they don't provide you with many advantages. Try switching to more complex whole-grain foods like quinoa, brown rice, and bread. These are more gratifying since they take longer for your body to digest. Complex carbohydrates are also included in a variety of fruits and vegetables, such as spinach and cauliflower. As alcohol contains calories with few nutritional benefits, it should be avoided or consumed in moderation. It can also weaken your self-control, slow down your metabolism, and impede judgment.

4. Carry out strength training activities three to four times per week. Plan 30- to 45-minute training sessions where you work your upper body one day and your lower body the next. To give your muscles a chance to recover and relax, perform your strength training activities every other day. When lifting, be careful to pick a weight with which you are at ease. The weight should be high enough to be tough while still being low enough for you to complete all of your reps. When you begin to feel comfortable with your regimen, increase the weight and reps.

5. Select workout plans that concentrate on a certain muscle group. Choose a different muscle group to concentrate on throughout your workout each day that you strength train. This strengthens every muscle in your body and keeps certain ones from being overly exhausted. Stretch the muscles you utilized throughout your workout afterward to avoid tension and improve flexibility.

Try performing barbell squats, leg presses, and deadlifts to strengthen your legs.[19] Practice dumbbell rows, pull-ups, and lateral raises to tone your chest and back. Practice wood chops, Russian twists, and sit-ups to strengthen your core muscles.

6. Exercise your heart five to six times per week. Do cardio exercises daily to maintain your tone. To burn calories and form healthy habits, try going for a jog, using a treadmill, or riding a bike. Try to complete 30 to 40 minutes of cardio each time you work out. Give yourself at least 1 day of rest each week to allow your body to rest. It's okay to work out with both cardio and strength equipment on the same day.

7. Enroll in a fitness class to participate in exercises with others. You can enroll in exercise classes at many recreation centers. Find out whether there is a free class session available for a class you are interested in, such as Zumba, CrossFit, or kickboxing. Once you locate one you like, enroll in the class so you may socialize while exercising. You might be able to discover comparable exercise plans online if you don't want to enroll in a class.

8. Yoga can assist you in toning your body. You may maintain your flexibility and increase your muscle endurance by practicing yoga. Start by practicing some basic postures for 15 to 30 minutes to get acclimated to the positions. Add more challenging postures to your program if you begin to feel comfortable in them. To follow along with a virtual instructor, watch videos online.

Chapter 6

The best exercises for building your trainable muscles and what they do.

The Ultimate Muscle Groups Guide & How To Train Them Best.

There are over 650 unique muscles in the human body, but you don't need to memorize them all to perfect weight training. Less is sometimes more. That's why we've reduced it to just eleven easy-to-remember muscle types. You'll also find the best muscle-group-specific suggestions culled from cutting-edge science, world-class instructors, and practical real-world experience. Follow the tips in this article to develop a fit, balanced physique while lowering your chance of injury.

Why Is Muscle Anatomy Important?

Why is understanding the various human muscle groups and their functioning crucial for your fitness? To begin, recognizing the major muscle groups is necessary if you want to build or select safe and effective training regimens. Simply said, avoiding muscular imbalances requires a fundamental understanding of muscle anatomy. Achieving overall muscle group balance is essential for excellent posture, injury avoidance, optimal function, and, of course, a solid body. That means that if you don't understand the major muscle groups and their functioning, the programs you design or choose may be unproductive or even dangerous.

Applying muscle group knowledge can also help you appear better. Old-school, drug-free bodybuilders from the 1940s and 1950s may have been the first to recognize this, but it applies equally to men and women today. So, if you want to reach your best physical potential, you'll need to include muscle anatomy knowledge into your training regimen.

Unfortunately, several sources confound the subject of muscle types. Most texts on the subject will give you a headache rather than information you can use during your next workout. Continue reading to learn the secrets to faster improvement, fewer injuries, and your finest body yet.

Glutes

Your gluteus maximus is the largest muscle in your body and one of the most significant for athletic performance and appearance. The gluteus medius and gluteus minimus, like their big brother gluteus maximus, start in the pelvis and insert into the femur. Your gluteal muscles are some of the strongest in your body. They are used in heavy or explosive compound actions such as deadlifts, squats, and sprints.

Furthermore, the benefits of glute exercise go beyond just utilitarian. According to studies, males find women with small waists and large buttocks particularly attractive. A male predilection for curvier buttocks appears to be increasing with time. Although there has been less research into women's preferences, it is not a secret that many women feel the same way males do. If you have any doubts about the social benefits of glute training, ask some of the women in your life if they find shapely glutes attractive.

Life is much more than aesthetics, yet who can resist enhanced athleticism and an amazing appearance? Fortunately, men and women alike can obtain strong, healthy, and attractive glutes by following a few basic workout suggestions. Even if you don't care about your appearance, strengthening your glutes can help you age gracefully by reducing lower back pain and stretching your hip flexor muscles. Early evidence suggests that weak glutes may potentially contribute to knee pain.

That implies strengthening your glutes could help you avoid pain in more ways than one.

Glute Exercises That Work

Barbell or Smith machine hip thrusts, weighted glute bridges, and dumbbell Romanian deadlifts are all effective exercises for activating and building your glutes. Deep goblet squats with a kettlebell or dumbbell. Start mild to master the movements, then gradually increase the weight to all of them as you gain proficiency. As long as you use proper form, your glutes can withstand a lot of weight. Combine hip thrusts and glute bridges with squats and deadlifts, which are typical lower-body compound workouts, for the best results.

Although some people consider hip thrusts and glute bridges to be "isolation" exercises, they are nevertheless among the most efficient glute builders available. Hip thrusts and glute bridges can assist in activating your glutes before squats or deadlifts while executing them afterward delivers further glute stimulation. Try both and see which you prefer, or alternate between the two over time. Keep most of your glute training sets between 5-12 reps, but towards the end of your exercise, you can complete some "burnout" sets of 20-30+ reps.

Trapezius, Rhomboids, and Lats (back)
The muscles in your back, including your glutes, are important for both performance and posture. Driving, sitting at a desk, using a smartphone, and watching TV are all examples of modern lifestyles that

involve a lot of sitting and slouching. As a result, many people are prone to injury due to bad posture. The good news is that you may correct these disorders by properly training your back. When we say back, we mean anything between your neck and butt on the back of your body. And, as you may be aware, there are various muscle groups in that area.

Trapezius

Your trapezius muscle is shaped like a diamond. It runs from your skull's occipital bone down to your thoracic spine (mid-back), and it's in charge of moving your scapulae (shoulder blades) and supporting your arms. Many people are unaware that the trapezius muscles have middle and lower aspects in addition to the "upper traps," which are visible next to your neck from the front of your body.

Putting too much emphasis on the upper traps, such as with shrugs, can lead to shoulder impingement (a lack of space for the rotator cuff tendon in the shoulder joint, which can result in bone pressing the tendon and causing pain or tearing).

Rhomboids

Your rhomboids are the muscles that link your shoulder blades to your mid-back. Because they are virtually concealed beneath the trapezius, they are frequently weak and underutilized in many training programs. Rhomboid muscles retract and rotate your shoulder blades downward, which is necessary for excellent posture. As a result, strengthening your rhomboids is an excellent approach to counteract the detrimental consequences of sitting for hours each day.

Dorsi Latissimus Dorsi

Finally, the latissimus dorsi (or lats) are the largest muscles in your upper torso. They play an important role in vertical pulling actions and also help stabilize your upper body during horizontal pressing. These broad, flat, triangular muscles run from the mid-back to the lower back. People frequently confuse them with the smaller teres major and minor, which are located above the lats and closer to the shoulder joint.

Optimal Back Exercises

The majority of back exercises, but not all of them, include "pulling" actions. Here are a few instances:

-Cable seated high rope face pulls (middle and lower traps with optional external rotation).

-Rhomboids with sitting low rope or V-bar cable row.

-A one-arm dumbbell row while standing with support (20–30 degrees; rhomboids and lats).

-A 35–45 degree bent-over barbell row for the traps, rhomboids, lats, and lower back.

-Pull-ups and chin-ups, which work the major and minor lats and teres.

-Plate-loaded machine pull-downs as an alternative to pull-ups.

-Heavy half-rack deadlift from a height above the knee with a 1-2 second hold at the top (worked every back muscle in plenty).

Single-joint exercises are not included because they are ineffective for developing a strong back. But if you perform the aforementioned compound motions with proper form, you can isolate your traps, rhomboids, or lats.

Always practice proper form before attempting heavier weights. To maintain a good balance between pulling and pushing, it's also advisable to perform more volume for your back than your chest, which is the opposite of what most individuals do.

Chest

The muscles in your chest are important for pushing motions that are horizontal as well as for humerus (upper arm bone) control. Bodybuilders love the thick, fan-shaped pec major, but regardless of your objectives, strengthening your chest intelligently is a great idea. Along with the well-known pectoralis major ("pecs"), the serratus anterior and pectoralis minor also cooperate. The serratus muscles, which resemble fingers, are located on your ribcage beneath your pecs and armpits, whereas the pec minor is concealed below the pec major.

Optimal Chest Exercises

Since the chest is not a very difficult muscle area, it is recommended to train it with these straightforward exercises: Wide-grip, incline, push-ups, dips, and partial range of motion (ROM) chest press Cable flies (any version), bench press (all other varieties). Push-ups and dips have several advantages: they can be performed using only your body weight, they may be more "functional" in real life because they are closed-chain motions, and they engage stabilizers like your serratus, which lowers your chance of injury.

We also enjoy using Levels' incline partial ROM bench press to develop large, complete pecs, especially for taller people. Modify your range of motion to achieve it by lowering the barbell halfway to your chest rather than locking it out at the top. This technique adequately engages your pecs while keeping your shoulder at a safer angle. The other exercises can help you develop your pecs just as effectively as the flat, full-range-of-motion bench press, which is a staple of strength training across the globe. If you are drawn to bench pressing frequently, go for it, but make sure your form and shoulder health are impeccable.

Last but not least, after training with complex movements, cable flies are a fantastic technique to isolate your chest while performing more reps. Additionally, they keep the strain on the muscle throughout the rep, in contrast to conventional dumbbell flies.

Shoulders

Unlike any other muscle in your body, your shoulders are unique. Every upper body movement involves the glenohumeral (shoulder) joint, which is one of your body's most delicate joints. There are seven heads (distinct bundles of muscle fibers that give the muscle its appearance) in your deltoids, the meaty spherical muscles on either side of your collarbone. However, it's simplest to consider them as having anterior (front), lateral (side), and posterior (back) heads to choose single-joint exercises to isolate your delts.

Training your anterior deltoids enlarges the front of your shoulders, but working your rear delts gives your back depth. Additionally, when viewed from the front or the rear, working your lateral deltoids helps your shoulders appear wider.

The fastest way to increase power and improve function is to strengthen the muscles around your shoulder joint. Additionally, it can aid in emphasizing a thin waist visually, giving men and women a curvaceous appearance or a "V" shape.

Recommended Shoulder Exercises

It's impossible to raise weights without working your shoulders. They support all motions of the upper body as well as many of the lower body movements. But use the following compound and isolation exercises to highlight or strengthen your delts: standing overhead presses with a barbell, single or double kettlebells,

(Anterior deltoids) Plate front rise, Slow negative dumbbell lateral rise (2–3 seconds) (lateral deltoids), a 1-second hold at the top of a bent-over, single-arm dumbbell rear delt raise (posterior deltoids), Standing overhead presses (OHPs) are a traditional weight training exercise that work almost all of your body's muscles, making them particularly "functional." Fitness enthusiasts employed OHPs before bench presses were popular to assess their strength.

In addition, you just need a few free weights and a small amount of standing space to obtain a superb shoulder workout. First, try pounding your shoulders with a powerful compound pressing motion. To end the exercise, perform lighter, higher-volume sets of front, lateral, and rear delt lifts. You run the risk of suffering a serious injury like a rotator cuff tear or shoulder separation if you train through the pain.

Consider yourself fortunate to have received a warning if you experience pain while moving your shoulders, and pay attention to it. In the end, it's better to avoid the risk because other pushing and pulling motions can still stimulate your shoulders sufficiently.

Quadriceps

The four muscles that make up your quadriceps, sometimes known as "quads," are found on the front of your thighs and are responsible for extending your knees. The vastus lateralis, vastus medialis, vastus intermedius, and rectus femoris are those muscles. The rectus femoris flexes your hips as well as extending your knees.

The muscles of your quads originate on your femur and insert into the base of your patella (kneecap), except the rectus femoris, which originates on the iliac spine of your pelvis. it's a mistake to train your upper body and neglect your lower body.

It turns out that one of the best methods to improve your general health and look is by correctly training your lower body, especially your quads. Increasing anabolic hormones like testosterone and growth hormone, can even improve your outcomes for your upper body.

Recommended Quadriceps Exercises

Squats must be mentioned if discussing how to exercise your quads. Squats should always be a part of your routine unless you are utterly incapable of doing them, which is doubtful. How about security? The most recent generation of academics and trainers concur with the outdated notion that deep, hard squats are intrinsically hazardous for your knees.

Although you might have an undiscovered injury or poor form if you experience knee pain while squatting, this does not necessarily mean that squats are to blame. If nothing else, many individuals with ongoing discomfort or past injuries can still squat safely and painlessly while using smaller weights. Try the exercises listed below to see which one you like best:

Goblet squats with dumbbells or kettlebells, Squats with two kettlebells while holding them in the rack position, Barbell back squats and box squats Leg presses, Split squats, or Bulgarian split squats. Barbell front squat. Machine hack squat. You can occasionally switch up your main squat movement, but for optimal results, stick with one for a few months at a time.

The most suitable exercises for beginners are goblet squats, double kettlebell squats, and box squats. Alternatively, if you don't feel comfortable doing squats, find a knowledgeable instructor or stick to machine hack squats and leg press variations.

What about extending your legs? This isolated exercise strains your knee joint and anterior cruciate ligament (ACL), and it doesn't have the same hormone-boosting effects as compound exercises. Leg extensions may also harm the cartilage in the knee joints, according to many knowledgeable trainers, even if there is no scientific agreement on the subject. So, if you value having good knees, skip them.

If you want to go beyond the fundamentals and boost the volume of your quad workout, split squats and variations like Bulgarian split squats are a preferable choice.

Hamstrings

On the rear of your legs, your hamstrings are responsible for flexing your knees and extending your hips. The hamstrings also receive little attention, much like a lot of the muscles on the back of the body. It's unfortunate because concentrating on them is essential for fitness and injury avoidance. Despite being around half the size of your quads, your hamstrings are a member of your posterior chain, along with your calves, glutes, and other muscles in the back of your body. The most crucial muscle group for athletic performance may be the posterior chain.

Too much quad exercise without proper hamstring training is very prevalent and can increase the risk of knee pain and injury by almost five times.

In addition, quad-hamstring imbalances increase the chance of suffering an ACL tear. Maintaining the proper balance between your thigh muscles is essential for female athletes because they already have 2–8 times more risk of suffering an ACL tear than male athletes. Both men and women are susceptible to muscle rips in their weak, tight hamstrings, especially when they perform sprinting or other explosive actions.

The ideal hamstring exercise.

The best exercises for developing better, stronger hamstrings are listed below:

Deadlifts (with a barbell, hex bar, or another full range-of-motion variation), Romanian deadlifts with dumbbells, glute-ham raises (using a machine or your body weight), and lying machine leg curls. Start slow and easy if you've never worked your hamstrings to prevent tearing a muscle.

Compound exercises are essential for strengthening the hamstrings, as they are for all muscle groups (such as deadlifts and their variations). Because it's generally not a good idea to pre-fatigue your hamstrings with single-joint actions, perform them before glute-ham raises or leg curls. Additionally, releasing tight hamstrings, static stretching after lifting, and dynamic mobility exercises (stretching or warm-up exercises that entail actively moving the joint or limb through its range of motion) before your workout can improve your function. However, it's typically advised to avoid excessive static stretching before training because it can impair strength and explosiveness for up to 24 hours.

Calves

Your femur is where your calves begin, and they join the Achilles tendon there. They are made up of the soleus and gastrocnemius muscles. Resistance exercise for your calves is essentially optional if you're an athlete. These muscles get good functional exercise whenever you practice or play your sport since you use them anytime you jump or move your feet. However, bodybuilders and others who train exclusively for aesthetic reasons will benefit the most from calf exercises.

Optimal Calf Exercises

The largest predictor of how your calves look is the insertion point, or the point where your calf muscle meets your Achilles tendon, and you cannot change genetics.

A calf muscle with a very high insertion point is around the size of a tennis ball, whereas a low insertion point typically produces massive, well-shaped calves with little effort. However, to make the most of what you're working with, you can do the exercises listed below:

Standing one-legged calf raises on a step while using body weight or a dumbbell for additional resistance, finishing with a two-second static hold and squeeze, Using a leg press machine, elevate your legs in the air while keeping your knees straight. Leg press machine with 30-degree knee angle bent-leg calf raise, 3-second stretch at the bottom, and 90-degree knee angle bent-leg sitting calf raise.

When your knees are bent, your gastrocnemius contracts the most, and when your knees are straight, your soleus contracts the most. To properly work both muscles, you should blend workouts using bent and straight knees.

Calves, tempo changes, volume ranges, and repetitions. Stretch holds between reps, static top holds, and tempo variety appear to be the exercises that benefit calves the most. These methods are part of the suggested calf exercises we listed above.

However, why may calves differ from other muscles in terms of changing the rep pace? One explanation could be that when the stretch-shortening cycle (SSC), which allows you to jump explosively, moves the strain to your Achilles tendon, it can take credit away from your calves. You'll need to outwit the SSC using pauses or slow negatives (that is, emphasizing the eccentric phase of the repeat by slowing it down to 2-3 seconds or more) because training calves explosively doesn't activate them as well as it does most muscles. Every time you train your lower body, you should include two or three calf exercises with a few sets each. If you want faster results, try shocking them with 12 to 15 total sets throughout each lower-body workout for a few weeks or longer.

Furthermore, calves typically grow the fastest with a variety of exercises. Try varying your rep ranges between 5 and 30 or more times.

Triceps

Want arms with muscle? Start with your triceps since they make up two-thirds of your upper arm's muscle mass. This three-headed muscle is extremely powerful and explosive, thus athletes and strength enthusiasts place a high priority on it. The long, lateral, and medial heads make up the triceps. Although their main function is to stretch your elbow, the lengthy head also helps to stabilize your shoulder.

Recommended Triceps Exercises

You may be sure that these triceps exercises will increase your strength, power, and definition. They are one-arm dumbbell overhead triceps extensions, inclined overhead two-handed dumbbell triceps extensions, overhead two-handed rope cable extensions with low pulleys, narrow-grip dips, reverse-grip barbell bench presses, barbell floor presses, and one-arm dumbbell overhead triceps extensions. Dips, reverse-grip bench press, and floor press all permit heavyweight and a comparatively extensive range of motion. The goal of these workouts is to use a complex movement to overload the triceps.

In contrast, overhead triceps isolation exercises are the ideal way to highlight the longest head of your triceps. Stretching and shoulder flexion work together to activate the long head, which causes amazing muscle growth. Additionally, avoid certain triceps exercises if they cause elbow pain in favor of ones that don't. Never disregard pain while moving; it's always a warning sign that needs attention.

Biceps

Your biceps have two heads: a short head and a long head. They work in opposition to the triceps and are in charge of elbow flexion. But try making these exercises a regular part of your routine before going down the rabbit hole of curling. Narrow-grip chin-ups, standing barbell curls, cross-body hammer curls to the level of the pecs (one arm at a time, switching reps by reps), and reverse-grip EZ bar curls are other exercises you can do.

Narrow-grip chin-ups are a complex exercise that offers more practical fitness applications than curls while heavily overloading your biceps.

And for good reason, standing barbell curls are the go-to exercise for biceps isolation. All you had to do was chin-ups and barbell curls for years to get bigger, stronger biceps.

Although the brachialis is largely out of sight and out of mind, giving it some attention will help you strengthen and round up your upper arms. The greatest brachialis workouts include reverse-grip EZ curls and cross-body hammer curls.

Abs

The rectus abdominis, inner and outer obliques, and the secret transversus abdominis make up your abs. Your lumbar spine is flexed, rotated, and stabilized by them all. One of the most sought and misunderstood exercise objectives is developing six-pack abs.

A smaller waist is not a result of training your abs, with one exception that we'll discuss shortly. Instead, spot reduction through ab exercises doesn't work effectively for fat loss. In actuality, bulking up your waist by doing hundreds of crunches might help you develop your abs. Additionally, a blockier waist is the visible outcome if your abs are covered in a regular amount of body fat. The vast majority of crunchers want the exact opposite of that! Crunches also cause your spine to flex, which could make your posture worse and raise your risk of back injury. Your back may potentially become injured by ab movements that rotate or twist.

What then is the key to ab training? Focus on function and injury avoidance when exercising your abs. This strategy is perfect for the great majority of gym members when combined with an awesome exercise routine and a healthy diet. A healthy diet is essential if you're intent on seeing your abs. In actuality, ripped abs begin in the kitchen.

When your abdominal muscles start to show, you could choose to add some more crunches to "fine-tune" what you see. What about the abdominal exercises that reduce waistline size? Theoretically, anything that engages your transversus abdominis (TA) will cause your waist to get smaller. Your internal obliques are a thin sheet of muscle known as the TA. It is what enables you to draw your belly button inside, yet you can't see it. The TA compresses and holds your viscera (internal organs), as well as supporting your core. You might be able to somewhat reduce your waist by toning it up.

Excellent ab exercises

It makes sense to incorporate a few sets of crunches or other ab flexion exercises into your weekly program. A terrible idea is to perform tens of thousands of repetitions of any resistance training exercise per week. Nowadays, astute coaches and trainers give other ab actions more importance than flexion. Prioritizing your ab muscles' stabilizing (bracing and anti-rotation) functions above your spine-moving (flexion and rotation) patterns is the key to a healthy spine and excellent posture. The new hierarchy is as follows:

Flexion, Bracing, Anti-Rotation, and Rotation

Be aware that while anti-rotation refers to fighting rotation, bracing involves resisting flexion or extension. Exercises to develop a strong, healthy midsection include:

Pallof press (anti-rotational exercise, also known as rotation resistance), pushup posture plank (bracing), Reverse crunches on a slant board, and cable crunches while kneeling, Optional motions include hanging pikes, dragon flags, or other toes-to-bar flexion exercises, full contact barbell twists (rotations), and ab vacuums (or yoga's Nauli kriya) for TA activation.

Early on, focus mostly on bracing before introducing anti-rotation. Move on to flexion and eventually rotation once you've mastered those.

Additionally, when performing flexion motions, don't be afraid to load them up. It is far more efficient to build strong abs with difficult weights than to perform endless repetitions.

Hands and arms

You are only as strong as your grasp for the vast majority of tasks in the actual world. Consider the possibility that you could push or pull hundreds of pounds using a barbell with a 1.1-inch diameter and an even balance, but what about heavier objects?

There are three primary grip techniques you can practice: Crush grip, in which your fingers flex in the direction of your palms. Pinch grip, where your fingers and thumb flex inward. Support grip refers to the static holding of a heavy object in your hands during deadlifts, farmer's walks, or when lifting abrasive things like boulders. Additionally, by keeping your wrists stable and avoiding lower arm injuries, developing strong forearms might benefit your grip over time.

Best Exercises for the Grip and Arms

The only restriction on your grip exercises is your imagination, however, these are the greatest ones to start with Grippers (Crush or similar captains), Using one or two weight plates and a pinch grip,

rows or carries using a pinch grip carrying heavy loads, especially when using kettlebells, Deadlifts with an overhand grip and a heavy partial rack without straps (bonus: use a fat bar), pull-ups while holding onto a towel, martial arts gi, or another sturdy object (alter your grip between sets), reverse wrist curls, wrist curls, reverse-grip dumbbell curl with one arm Rubber band finger extension serves as a counterbalance to finger flexion movements and may aid with carpal tunnel syndrome symptoms.

At any time, you can incorporate grip exercises into your routine. For instance, keeping a gripper at your workplace enables you to practice your crush grasp all day long.

Final Reflections

You can maintain balance and avoid injuries if you have a rudimentary understanding of muscle anatomy. Remember that if you want a robust, healthy body, you need to concentrate on more than simply "mirror muscles." Abstraction from core and chest muscles can result in poor posture and possibly major injury.

Furthermore, when properly developed, muscles like your glutes, back, and hamstrings not only look beautiful but help balance out other muscles you may have been concentrating on too much. Prioritizing your recovery is essential for achieving results and avoiding injuries, along with wise training. Therefore, if you exercise vigorously, remember to consume adequate calories and use whey protein post-workout to speed up your body's healing processes.

Now that you're knowledgeable about the various muscle groups, it's time to focus on your areas of weakness, correct any imbalances, and boost your performance.

Chapter 7

Formulating training activities for building an amazing body.

While there is nothing wrong with adhering to a one-size-fits-all, cookie-cutter training routine, you'll achieve better results if you do so. With our detailed instructions, you may learn the fundamentals of program design. You may follow a variety of fantastic programs on Fitness Volt. Simply pick the one you prefer the look of, print it off or download it, and complete the task. Although you'll still need to exercise regularly, eat healthfully, and get enough rest, we've done all the legwork for you in terms of planning. But there are drawbacks to following one of our regimens as well. To begin with, the author must create an exercise program for a group of people rather than just you. Exercises that you can't perform or don't enjoy may be included, and the program is unable to take into consideration your unique situation. For your present level of strength and fitness, the workout may be either too difficult or too simple. It could not even align with your training objectives. If you've worked out before, you could have the skills to analyze a program and then modify it to suit your needs. Exercisers with less training typically lack this ability.

You could pay a personal trainer or strength coach to create a customized training schedule for you. To find out what kind of plan you desire and require, a qualified trainer will ask you several questions. This requires spending money, though, and there is still no assurance that you'll come up with a good fitness schedule. Additionally, you'll have to repeat the procedure in a few months when your body adapts to your training, you stop seeing results, and you need a new strategy. We're going to provide you with the knowledge you need in this article so that you may design your custom routines. Just adhere to the directions listed below.

Step one: Choose your training objective.

Possibly the most important stage when beginning to construct your software is this one. It is what decides the kind of workout you will perform. You are fit for the types of workouts you conduct, according to the specificity principle. Therefore, your workout must be tailored to your objectives if you want to increase your strength, burn fat, or build muscle.

Specify in writing what you hope to achieve from your workout by taking a moment. Avoid trying to practice for many objectives at once; doing so makes

life more difficult than it needs to be and may even impede your training results. Choose the objective that is most important to you instead. This typically signifies one of the following for lifters:
muscular stamina

Increasing muscle mass

Strength

Power/speed

Remember that some of these objectives have a small overlap. Strength training will also develop muscle size and power while training for muscle size will increase strength and endurance.

Step 2: Select your rep range and rest intervals.

Every training objective has a particular rep range assigned to it. Determining your personal training objective is crucial for this reason. While exercising outside the recommended rep range for your objective will result in some progress, you'll perform better if you follow these recommendations.

objective of exercise Rep scale

Power and force1-5

Hypertrophy6-12

Endurance13-20

When deciding on your rep range, you have some leeway. For instance, you may perform sets of 4–8 if you want to increase both strength and size. Similar to this, you might concentrate on sets of 10-15 reps if you want to increase muscle size and endurance.

How long you should wait in between sets depends on your rep range as well. Generally speaking, you need to rest longer when using heavier weights and performing fewer reps per set. Because your central nervous system (CNS), which takes longer to recover than your muscles, is taxed by really intense strength training, this is the case. By training aim, the generally recognized rest intervals are as follows:

The objective of exercise time
Power and force to 5 min
1-2 minutes of hypertrophy
Endurance 30 to 60 sec.

Many programs also outline the amount of weight you should lift in relation to your 1RM, or one-repetition maximum. This can work, but it can also lead to issues when you're writing your program. To begin with, to prescribe a percentage of your 1RM, you must know it.

You could discover that some days you feel more powerful than others. These normal oscillations are not possible when you train at a fixed percentage of your 1RM. Instead of obsessing over 1RMs and percentages, focus instead on making sure you reach muscle failure within the confines of your selected rep range. You may need to experiment a little at first, but after about a week, you should establish your rhythm and identify the ideal weights to use. The approved 1RM percentages by training objective are as follows:

The goal for exercise %1RM
Strength and capability 85%>
67–85% hypertrophy
67% of the score is for endurance.

Step three: Pick a training split.

Your split defines how frequently you'll exercise each week as well as which muscle groups you'll train daily. There are many alternatives available, including body part splits, where you work out 1-2 muscle groups at once, the full body split, the upper body/lower body split, the push-pull split, and the push-pull split with the legs.

The ideal split will depend on how many days a week you can commit to working out. The greatest workout for you would definitely be a full-body split if you could only work out twice per week. Instead, you may employ a body part split if you can work out four, five, or even six times each week.

Step four:Choose your training volume.

Your planned number of sets each session, which might be high, moderate, or low, is referred to as your training volume. Generally speaking, you'll perform more sets the less your reps are. Therefore, you should anticipate performing more sets when performing sets of three reps as opposed to sets of 15 reps.How long you want to spend working out also affects the volume of your activity. You might deliberately perform fewer sets with each session if you don't have much time to train. However, you could want to perform additional sets if you have plenty of time to practice.

How many exercises you plan to include in each workout will also affect the number of sets you perform. You may perform a variety of exercises but only perform a few sets of each, or you could perform fewer activities but more sets.

To complete 15 sets, for instance, you may choose five different chest exercises and perform three sets of each, or you could perform just three exercises for the same number of sets.

In order to train the target body part from a number of perspectives, bodybuilders frequently include a wider variety of exercises per muscle group per workout. In contrast, people who exercise to build strength frequently perform fewer exercises but more repetitions of each activity. Every exercise in your routine doesn't have to be performed for the exact same amount of sets. The first few exercises should be your top priority, so you might find it preferable to perform more sets of those and less sets of the exercises toward the end of your program. Your energy is better utilized in this way.

Given that they are undoubtedly the "bigger bang" activity that will result in the majority of your gains, you can see from the example below that you'll be performing more sets of squats and leg presses than the other exercises.

5 sets of 5 repetitions for squats
4 sets of 8 repetitions on the leg press
3 sets of 10 repetitions of leg extensions
Leg curls: three sets of 10 repetitions
2 sets of 12 repetitions on the lunge

Whatever method you choose, your workout volume must match the amount of time you have to exercise. Determine how long your workout will last, and then find out how many sets you can do. For instance, your set should last roughly 105 seconds if you are training for hypertrophy, performing ten reps every set with a 60-second break in between each. You have enough time to do approximately 34 sets per session if you schedule a 60-minute workout. You can probably fit 25 to 28 sets into an hour-long workout if you take into account the time it takes to set up between exercises.

Naturally, your set count will be significantly lower or your workout will need to be much longer if you are strength training and need to rest three minutes in between sets. Although it's not necessary to fit as many sets into your workout as you can, it will be helpful to be aware of your top limit.

Step five:Choose an exercise.

You can pick from hundreds or even thousands of different strength training activities. However, in general, every activity can be classified as an isolation or compound exercise. Multiple muscle groups and two or more joints are used in compound workouts. Squats, deadlifts, bench presses, pull-ups and pull-downs, shoulder presses, and rows are a few examples.

You can lift high weights during compound workouts, which is beneficial for increasing your muscular size, strength, and power. Due to the fact that compound workouts frequently incorporate or mimic common actions, they are also thought to be more functional. Less muscle groups are used and only one joint moves at a time during isolation exercises. They work well for localized hypertrophy and endurance but less well for strength and power development. Dumbbell curls, cable flyes, triceps kickbacks, and calf raises are a few examples of solitary exercises.

Your program should contain more compound exercises than isolation exercises for practically all training objectives. Compound exercises let you get more exercise for your time while also speeding up your routine. Squats, for instance, work almost all of the muscles in your lower body. Leg extensions, Leg curls, Hip extensions, Hip abductions, Hip adductions, Lower back extensions, and Planks are all isolation exercises that can target the same muscles.

But that doesn't mean that isolation workouts are useless. Compound exercises are just frequently a better tool for the job. After performing your chosen compound exercises, you can "finish off" a main muscle with isolation exercises, or you can use them to target minor muscles that might require more attention. Compound versus isolation exercise ratios are not predetermined for each program. If you only do compounds, according to certain training professionals, nothing can go wrong!

Although they are not entirely necessary, isolation exercises should only make up around 20% of your total training volume in order to get the most out of your time and resources. Choose 1-2 isolation exercises in addition to 2-3 compound exercises for each muscle group you wish to train. Keep in mind that you can perform less sets of each exercise the more exercises you perform. On the other hand, if you pick fewer exercises, you can perform more sets of each activity.

Step six: workout sequencing

Now that you know the rep range you'll use, the number of sets you'll perform during a workout, the amount of time you need to rest in between sets, the body areas you'll train when, and the exercises you'll perform, you can plan your program accordingly.

Put those exercises in a sensible order as your next task. Generally speaking, it's ideal to progress from complex, heavy-weight compound workouts to simpler, lighter isolation exercises. This maximizes your energy, and when you exhaust yourself, your workout will get simpler. For instance, you might perform your exercises in the following order on your back day: deadlifts, pull-ups, seated rows, single-arm rows, and straight arm pulldowns.

Obviously, what one person deems difficult may be simple to another, so this phase is subject to some personal interpretation. But if you finish your workout unable to do the exercises you selected, you may have overexerted yourself because you saved the hardest exercises for last.

The impact of one exercise on your performance of the following should also be taken into account when choosing the order of the exercises. Back extensions should not be performed before to deadlifts as this will result in a weary lower back during the deadlift. Similar to this, you would perform worse if you trained your triceps before bench presses or overhead presses.

Step seven: Consider the progression

If you followed the preceding instructions, you should now have a solid training plan to adhere to. You'll be aware of the exercises you'll do, the sets and reps you'll do, and the muscle areas you'll be working on each day.

No matter how effective your program (ideally!) is, it only has a short shelf life because, after you've used it a few times, it won't be as effective as when you first started.Your body adjusts to any training fairly fast, therefore if you want to keep improving your endurance, strength, or muscle size, your workout Must be progressive. To that end, you must consider how you will make your software harder over the next few weeks as you are developing it. Increasing the weight, performing more reps per set, performing more sets, taking shorter breaks between sets, and other options are available. Using more difficult workouts, Include a training program.

To sustain your improvement, you usually don't need to make significant adjustments to your workout. To avoid training plateaus, constantly plan for development. If you remain with the same routine for too long, though, your progress will abruptly stop.

Step eight: Review and make any required revisions.

What seems nice on paper sometimes doesn't work out so well in practice. If your software isn't entirely flawless the first time you execute it, don't be alarmed. After your workout, reflect on what went particularly well and what wasn't as successful as you had intended. Make adjustments as necessary. For instance, you might have worked out for 90 minutes instead of the hour you had intended. Or you might discover that you were simply too exhausted to complete the last few workouts. Maybe the order of the exercises wasn't exactly perfect. When you begin creating your own programs, all of this is very normal and a necessary part of the learning process.

Make changes to your workout so that it goes more smoothly the next time.

Hopefully, you'll learn from these errors and avoid repeating them.

Building Your Program

Creating your own workouts requires both art and talent. Like any difficult endeavor, it can initially appear like a drawn-out and even convoluted procedure, but the more frequently you perform it, the easier it becomes. Additionally, if you persist, you'll discover how to design training plans that are better suited to your requirements and objectives.In other words, you will be rewarded if you create your own workout! There is nothing wrong with adhering to a plan made by someone else, but if it wasn't made especially for you, it might not be a perfect fit.

Follow the eight phases listed above as you construct your software from the ground up. Then, repeat the process for practice while devising a new routine. The more times you use this strategy, the more proficient you will become. Have fun with program design and try out various strategies. Every program you create should be saved; even if you don't want to use it right away, it might still work perfectly in the future.

Chapter 8:

How to design a diet that changes your body.

Even the most expertly designed program would be a complete waste of time without the proper nourishment. The majority of great athletes will agree that proper nutrition is more than half the battle and will prioritize it at least as much as their training regimen.

Three things are necessary for training progress: the training stimulus, restful sleep, and nourishing food. Of these three, nutrition comes out on top since it offers the assistance growing muscles require and permits adequate training intensity in the weight room. Lack of dietary information is frequently the main factor in why people's training attempts do not succeed. Bodybuilders frequently discover that their food intake is either insufficient for muscle growth or excessively high in the wrong nutrients. Consistency is the key to eating well for sports objectives.

Variety is vital, but if you want to see long-lasting effects, it's better to adhere to one diet than to vary your approach. Many bodybuilders alternate weeks of high and low-carbohydrate diets. Or they can get two days every week where they can do whatever they want. This is a bad notion since it will take the body two days to become used to a new eating routine, and even then, it will be difficult for the athletes to continue their diet after a two-day break.

The 12-week training cycle suggested in this book can be used in conjunction with the 1-week nutrition plan contained in it to assist lean mass growth and fat loss. It has the ideal balance of proteins, lipids, and carbohydrates to provide you with unmatched gains. But you have to be reliable.

So what exactly are carbohydrates, lipids, and proteins? The majority of us are aware of what these are, yet a startlingly high percentage are unaware. The question, "How many grams of protein are there in a banana?" was recently heard. We shall now focus on the fundamentals of nutrition with that question in mind. The "big three" nutrients—protein, carbs, and fats, or macronutrients—are typically mentioned when discussing nutrients in relation to health, fitness, and bodybuilding.

The micronutrients, vitamins, and minerals, are also crucial since they supply the essential building blocks for healthy metabolic activity. They aid in the absorption of the three macronutrients and are themselves present in variable amounts of proteins, lipids, and carbs. Following is a description of the macronutrients. Your diet will be based on the macronutrients because they give you the energy and building blocks you need to grow. They include the following things.

Protein

Protein, which has 20 amino acids and four calories per gram, is said to be the most important nutrition for bodybuilders since it helps develop muscles and every cell in our bodies (which total over 100 trillion cells). Your exercise efforts won't result in any more muscle gain if you don't consume enough protein. Marathon runners, who often eat very little protein and train for long periods of time, are a good example of how too little protein can lead to muscle wastage. There are 20 amino acids in proteins, of which 10 are necessary and 10 are non-essential. Since amino acids are the building blocks of proteins, they influence the quality of a particular protein source.

The non-essential kind can be produced by the body, but the necessary kind needs to be consumed as part of a healthy, balanced diet. For people looking to gain muscle, such as those reading this piece, food sources deficient in the required amino acids are consequently a bad choice. This diet plan emphasizes foods with a high biological value (HBV) of proteins.

The term "high biological value" refers to complete proteins that are rich in the key amino acids needed to develop muscle. When lifting heavy weights for extended periods of time, the muscle tissue is really subjected to microtrauma (little tears that must be mended), which is why these amino acids are so crucial.

It takes enough protein to rebuild the muscle to higher levels after this micro-trauma, which is effectively the breakdown of muscle tissue. With the appropriate protein intake and enough training stimulus, as described in this section, the muscles should make up for it by growing bigger and stronger in anticipation of the next workouts. Only by replacing protein levels do they adapt to the imposed stress. To enable the creation of new muscle tissue, muscles require an ongoing supply of protein.

The precise amount of protein that a hard-training strength/bodybuilding athlete should eat has been the subject of heated discussion over the years. Lower levels are felt by some. For example, 5 grams per pound of body weight per day is sufficient for repair and recovery needs. For a 180-pound trainee, this would translate to 90 grams of protein, which could be split up into three 30-gram meals per day. While some people still believe in this percentage today, most understand that a bodybuilder who trains hard, or even a leisure lifter, requires at least twice as much, if not more. For certain people, the protein intake per pound of body weight can reach two to three grams.

One to 1.5 grams of high biological value protein per pound of body weight is excellent and must be attained for the specific aims of persons reading this article. The diet described below will offer one to 1.5 grams of protein per pound of body weight for people of varying weights. This diet is designed so that you will get 205 to 235 grams of high-quality protein per day spread out over six meals, each of which contains about 35 to 41 grams of protein (including protein from other sources like oatmeal and whole wheat bread), depending on your training goals of gaining unheard-of muscle size while losing fat.

For speedier muscle recovery on training days, an additional 20–30 grams of protein will be ingested after the weight training session, bringing the total protein intake for that day to about 250–255. Six smaller meals rather than three larger ones will speed up metabolism and aid in fat burning. Additionally, the smaller protein servings throughout the day will help with muscle building because the muscles will get all the amino acids they require for growth throughout the day rather than at certain, less ideal times. This diet contains the ideal quantity of protein for someone weighing 205 pounds or less. People who weigh more will need more protein, thus an additional protein shake (providing about 30 grams of protein per day) can be consumed.

The finest foods for training are those with the highest biological value proteins, such as eggs, poultry, fish, milk, and steak because they contain all of the essential amino acids in the proper balance that humans need for survival.

You can also use protein powders, particularly those with whey bases (whey is the fastest-absorbing, highest biological quality powder available), to consume enough of this crucial vitamin. To reiterate, one to 1.5 grams of protein per pound of body weight is ideal for people who exercise frequently and hard. Therefore, a 175-pound individual would take in between 175 and 262 grams of protein per day. Although 175 grams is acceptable, it is recommended to fall between this number and 262, for instance, approximately 230 grams.

As the body's primary nutrient for repair, protein will aid in our efforts to gain muscle. Reduce your body fat since it speeds up your metabolism more than any other food. Keep from feeling hungry, which will stop you from seeking unhealthy foods. Boost tissue repair. boost immune performance. build vital hormones and enzymes. When carbohydrates are not available, give energy. Conserve your lean muscular mass.

Eggs, whey protein supplements, milk, cottage cheese, chicken, fish, and steak are some examples of protein sources.

Carbohydrates

Carbohydrates are the main energy source for all human movement, but protein is the food that serves as the body's "building block." Carbohydrates, which also provide four calories per gram, combine with protein to ensure growth as a result of resistance training. Consuming the proper amount of protein may have little impact on muscle building if there isn't a strong workout stimulus.

One can train to their maximum ability when they consume carbohydrates. Numerous types of carbohydrates exist, and each one, when consumed in the right amounts at the right times, helps grow muscle. Following is a description of each of the two types of carbs included in the diet recommended in this book.

Various Carbohydrates

The number one workout fuel source in our regimen is complex carbs, so named because they take longer to break down and keep us going longer. The two divisions of complex carbohydrates(starchy and fibrous)are collectively referred to as "healthy carbohydrates".

Potatoes, rice, cereals, spaghetti, pasta, and wholemeal bread are all considered to be in the starchy category. Brown rice, whole grain bread, and jacket potatoes make up the starchy carbohydrate portion of this diet because they have more fiber, which promotes weight loss and good health in general.

Asparagus, broccoli, cauliflower, onions, and spinach are examples of fibrous carbohydrates that often give a diet more volume without adding too many calories. Since they contain a range of vitamins and minerals, they are frequently categorized as the more nutritionally dense of the carbohydrate types. They are quite significant and shouldn't be disregarded just for this reason. The diet recommended here primarily consists of broccoli to increase metabolic rate and burn more body fat while delivering the micronutrients for better metabolic function throughout the body.

Basic Carbohydrates

Simple sugar carbs lack the natural nutrients included in complex and fibrous carbohydrates. These carbohydrates include sugar in all of its forms, milk, honey, chocolate, and cakes. Given that these nutrients aid in the metabolism of carbs, simple carbohydrates that do not contain them will be more easily transformed into, and stored as, fat. Additionally, simple sugar carbs frequently contain other chemicals that hinder muscle growth and lead to ill health. Additionally, they frequently raise insulin levels, which causes them to be transformed into fat. When excessive levels of insulin are released into the bloodstream, it uses all available energy (often in the form of circulating carbohydrates), which makes us feel exhausted.

One of the things we're attempting to prevent with this diet is that these carbohydrates are typically subsequently deposited as body fat. For people wanting to reduce weight, simple sugar carbs are frequently seen as the biggest possible issue. Apples, raspberries, melons, and oranges are examples of simple carbs that are low in sugar and a healthier alternative. These should occasionally be used in place of sugars in this diet.

Since one of the main objectives of this program is to reduce body fat levels, complex carbohydrates (both starchy and fibrous) are stressed because of their sustaining nature (providing longer-lasting energy for intense training sessions) and because they will not result in the rapid accumulation of fat as would the insulin-spiking simple carbohydrates. Simply carbs are mentioned less because, in moderation, they can help with training results. For quick energy replenishment, the liver and muscles both have the capacity to store carbohydrates for later usage as fuel. They are crucial for maintaining gut health and removing waste.

Brown rice, oatmeal, whole-wheat bread, potatoes, sweet potatoes, whole-wheat pasta, broccoli, spinach, bananas, oranges, and strawberries are all good sources of carbohydrates.

Fats

Similar to carbs, fats in all of their forms are an energy source. According to most estimations, unlike carbs, they won't provide energy in an optimum form and, at nine calories per gram, if consumed in excess, will almost certainly be stored as fat. From a health perspective, it is known that fats play a role in obesity and heart disease. All fats are not created equal, though. There are good and bad fats, and the diet recommended in this manual mainly includes the good kind.

Given that every cell in our body is made up of a fatty layer (the cell membrane), which aids in that cell's normal functioning, the right kind of fats in the right amounts will actually be beneficial to health. The cell membrane is the area of the cell that permits the entry of amino acids, carbohydrates, and other vital metabolites like lips (or fats), as well as for each cell's best function and waste product disposal.

Poor Fats

These fats, which include saturated and trans fats, are to blame for the unfavorable impacts on health that fat is so frequently associated with. In animal products such as meat, seafood, whole-milk dairy products like cheese, milk, ice cream, poultry skin, and egg yolks, saturated fats are present and solid at room temperature. They are major causes of heart disease because they raise blood cholesterol levels and obesity because they provide too many calories, which are more easily stored as fat.

Having said that, it has been demonstrated that a very tiny quantity of saturated fat can aid in the creation of testosterone, which results in increases in muscle mass and decreases in body fat. As this diet will demonstrate (a relatively tiny quantity of saturated fat will come from various animal sources), it's all about finding the correct balance.

When hydrogen is added to vegetable oil to extend its shelf life, a process known as hydrogenation takes place, producing trans fats as a byproduct. Commercial products often include trans fat, which will hinder your training and health if you consume it. Trans fat is added to products to increase longevity. It is not an essential fat, so the diet plan presented in this guide fully omits it.

Ideal Fats

The two types of healthy fats are polyunsaturated (found in vegetable oils, sunflower, cottonseed, and fish oils) and monounsaturated (found in natural foods like almonds, avocados, olive oil, grape-seed oil, corn oil, and canola oil). Polyunsaturated fat, which comes in its omega-three form, has a wider range of advantages over saturated fat, including the capacity to significantly reduce inflammation (great for the recovery process following exercise), inhibit the growth of cancer cells, and enhance brain function. Omega-three fish oil (discussed in the supplement section) is a natural choice for anyone who lifts weights because it has been demonstrated to significantly reduce muscle inflammation while also strengthening joints for bodybuilders. Monounsaturated fat also has some fantastic advantages, therefore it shouldn't be disregarded.

Benefits of good fats.

Olive oil, which is included in this program as the main fat component along with the polyunsaturated fish oil, is a crucial element of the much-lauded Mediterranean diet. Olive oil is known to thin the blood, enhance general health, and boost bodybuilding exercise outcomes. One important thing to keep in mind about so-called bad fats is that they can be found in many packaged foods and the majority of the animal meats are used in this diet. Trim any visible fat off chicken and steak, and choose water-packed tuna over oil-based to avoid the extra calories they deliver. Fats aid in our regular development and growth. The energy that is concentrated is found primarily in fat.

absorb specific vitamins (such as carotenoids, vitamins A, D, E, and K), provide the organs some padding, keep cell membranes intact, and Give food flavor, constancy, and stability.

Dietary Guidelines for Developing a Hard, Lean Body in 12 Weeks

The diet in the following plan is well-balanced in terms of proteins, carbohydrates, and fats, and it also contains important vitamins and minerals that will help you build muscle and perform better. To help you get the most out of the training regimen offered, this sample plan will define the ideal ratio of each macronutrient.

Food selections can be changed to a comparable product (described in the macronutrient overview), but for quality gains, the quantity and frequency of meals must remain constant throughout the course of the 12-week period. The amount of protein and complex carbohydrates that a larger individual training for maximum muscle size should consume can be changed; a smaller person training for moderate size would require a little less. Most persons starting the 12-week training program should be able to eat according to the diet as it is.

It must be emphasized that the following meal plan is merely an illustration of what one would eat on an average day. It does have a solid balance of nutrients, but its focus is on developing a muscular, athletic physique. The normal individual will naturally employ a diet lower in overall calories and macronutrients (bodybuilders, by virtue of the enormous demands they make on their bodies, are not average and need more nutrition).

Again, for the duration of the 12-week training program, the following one-week diet must be followed every week. The same meals should be consumed every day, however, for variety's sake, some food groups can be substituted (see the explanation of the macronutrients above). Keep in mind that the body benefits from consistency in nourishment. It will be the exercise that alters in order to force increases in muscle size and fat loss. About 37.5% of this diet's calories come from protein, 47.5 % from carbohydrates, and 15% come from fat.

Detailed Diet

Monday

Meal 1: 1 cup of oatmeal, 1 apple, 7 egg whites, 1 tablet of vitamins, 1 teaspoon of fish oil, and 2 glasses of water

Meal 2: Brown rice (1 cup), 1 serving of cottage cheese, and 2 glasses of water

Meal 3: Tuna (1 sandwich), 2 glasses of water

Meal 4: Brown rice (1 serve), 1 chicken, Olive oil (1 teaspoon), two glasses of water

Meal 5: 1 baked potato, 150 g of steak, 1 cup of broccoli, and 2 glasses of water.

Meal 6: Three egg whites, one protein shake

Tuesday

meal: 1 cup of oatmeal, 1 apple, 7 egg whites, 1 tablet of vitamins, and 1 teaspoon of fish oil. (2 glasses) of water

Meal 2: Tuna (1 sandwich), 2 glasses of water

Meal 3 consists of one serving each of cottage cheese, brown rice, water, and olive oil.

Meal 4: Brown rice (1 serve), 1 chicken breast (2 glasses) of water

Meal 5: Fish (300 g), 1 cup of broccoli, 1 baked potato

Meal 6: Protein shake, three egg whites

Wednesday

Meal 1 cup of oatmeal, 1 apple, 7 egg whites, 1 tablet of vitamins, and 1 teaspoon of fish oil.

Meal 2: Chicken, 1 cup of brown rice, and 2 glasses of water

Meal 3: Tuna (1 sandwich), 2 glasses of water

Meal 4: Chicken (1), Brown Rice (1), Olive Oil (1), Water (2)

Meal 5: 1 baked potato, 150 g steak, 1 cup broccoli, and 2 glasses of water.

Meal 6: Three egg whites, one protein shake

Thursday

Meal: 1 cup of oatmeal, 1 apple, 7 egg whites, 1 tablet of vitamins, 1 teaspoon of fish oil, and 2 glasses of water.

Meal 2: Tuna (1 sandwich), 2 glasses of water.

Meal 3: Brown rice (1 cup), 1 serving of cottage cheese, and 2 glasses of water.

Meal 4: Chicken (1), Brown Rice (1), Olive Oil (1), Water (2).

Meal 5: 1 baked potato, 250 g of steak, and 1 cup of broccoli.

Meal 6: Protein shake, 3 egg whites.

Friday

Meal: 1 cup of oatmeal, 1 apple, 7 egg whites, 1 tablet of vitamins, 1 tsp. fish oil, and 2 glasses of water.

Meal 2: Chicken, 1 cup of brown rice, and 2 glasses of water

Meal 3: Tuna (1 sandwich), 2 glasses of water

Meal 4: Chicken (1), Brown Rice (1), Olive Oil (1), Water (2).

Meal 5: 1 baked potato, 250 g of steak, and 1 cup of broccoli.

Meal 6: 250 g of cottage cheese

Saturday

Meal: Oatmeal (one cup), Apple, seven egg whites, vitamins (one tablet), fish oil (one teaspoon), and two glasses of water.

Meal 2: Chicken, 2 glasses of water, 1 cup of brown rice.

Meal 3: Tuna (1 sandwich), 2 glasses of water

Meal 4: Chicken (1), Brown Rice (1), Olive Oil (1), Water (2).

Meal 5: Fish, 1 baked potato, 1 cup of broccoli

Meal 6: Protein shake, 3 egg whites.

Sunday

Meal: 1 cup of oatmeal, 1 apple, 7 egg whites, 1 tablet of vitamins, 1 teaspoon of fish oil, and 2 glasses of water.

Meal 2: Chicken, 1 cup of brown rice, and 2 glasses of water

Meal 3: Two glasses of water, one serving of cottage cheese, and two pieces of whole wheat bread.

Meal 4: Chicken (1), Brown Rice (1), Olive Oil (1), Water (2)

Meal 5: 1 baked potato, 250 g steak, 1 cup broccoli, and 2 glasses of water.

Meal 6: Protein shake and three egg whites.

Tips for Eating Well

A well-balanced diet with the appropriate proportions of protein, fats, and carbohydrates is one thing; being sick from it is quite another. When looking for results in bodybuilding, the number one reason people don't advance is frequently nutrition-related. The following recommendations can be used as a guide for building muscle. You will achieve tremendous results if you use them consistently.

Regularly consume food all day long.
This diet is designed to enhance muscle building and fat loss by supplying essential nutrients at regular intervals. In addition to ensuring that your muscles receive the energy and growth nutrients they require to support continuous improvements, eating six equally spaced meals per day can also help you burn more

fat by boosting your metabolism (the rate at which your body burns calories). All meals must be consumed for this diet to be successful. If necessary, prepare your meals for the following day and plan your day in advance.

Make Sure You Have Enough Food.

It's crucial to have all the foods that make up your diet available when trying to eat all of your meals. Shop once a week with a list of all the foods you'll need for that week to help with this vital procedure. It ought to be simpler to organize your meals for any given day if you have all the foods listed in your diet, in the proper amounts. Having all the right foods on hand will also make it less likely for you to indulge in diet-busting foods, which frequently happens to people whose meals for the week have not been thoughtfully prepared.

Do Not Deceive

The ability to stick to the diet's recommended foods is another essential component. This involves abstaining from meals that will hinder your success in your diet. Cheat foods are ones that greatly exceed the recommended daily intake of sugar, trans fat, and saturated fat. Cakes, sweets, pizzas, cookies, and soft drinks like Coke fall into this category and should all be avoided at all costs. As your body gets used to eating the kinds of foods it was designed to eat, you may already not use these products, which is good.

Junk foods like the ones stated can obstruct the body's normal metabolic processes, which will have an adverse effect on muscle growth and fat burning. Eliminating obvious junk food doesn't mean you can't occasionally swap out a meal from this diet for one that is low in fat and simple sugar. This book includes two excellent dish suggestions to add some diversity to your program. The ideal would be one such supper every week.

Get some water

Ample water consumption throughout the day is a key element of this eating plan. Water is essential for the body's detoxification process and aids in the breakdown of food consumed, thus it should never be skipped, especially in humid weather.

Don't confuse hunger with thirst. Maintain Your Hydration.

Water is useful during exercise because it hydrates the muscles, keeping them strong and full, and ensures that nutrients are distributed freely throughout the body to support growth. Water also has a significant favorable impact on fat burning and promotes feelings of fullness, which reduces the desire to eat unhealthy foods.

Reduce your carb intake in the evening.
In this diet, evening carbohydrate intake is limited. The majority of people who consume a lot of carbohydrates in the evening typically struggle to lose weight and may even start gaining it. After the evening meal, which will follow the afternoon/evening workout, one must limit carbohydrates because they are easily converted to fat if not expended as energy.

Any type of carbohydrate, although excellent for energy, will cause weight gain if consumed at the incorrect time. It is also believed that eating carbohydrates in the evening can increase appetite, making cheating more likely. It is preferable to stick to protein in the evenings (as recommended by this diet plan).

Eat a meal at least two hours before exercising.

One of the secrets to a terrific workout is eating in the hours prior to training. Energy levels for training won't be adequate without enough nutrition, especially carbs. I've discovered that eating an hour prior to a workout will give you more energy than eating two hours beforehand. To determine which strategy suits you the best, try both. This eating plan is set up so that you get the most out of the pre-workout meal.

Afterwards, eat

Post-workout feedings are just as crucial as pre-workout nourishment. Post-workout nutrition will make sure that energy is restored and protein is delivered to the muscles at the time when they are most responsive to its beneficial effects, as opposed to the pre-workout meal, where energy generation is the planned objective. Many fitness professionals even go so far as to claim that the post-workout meal is the second-most crucial meal of the day, right behind breakfast.

The Value Of Post-Exercise Nutrition?

The muscles usually lose all of their glycogen stores after a vigorous workout, leaving a 30- to 45-minute window for replenishing. At this moment, protein is also quickly absorbed by the muscles. For effective outcomes, I personally advise, as mentioned in this program, combining a basic sugar formula with a portion of whey protein immediately following exercise (more on supplements below). The evening meal will follow this feeding in around 45 minutes.

Never skimp on breakfast.
It's become somewhat cliché to say that breakfast is the most important meal of the day, but with good reason: it's crucial to provide the body the nutrition it needs after what is basically an eight to ten-hour fast (thus the name breakfast; breakfast).

It is especially important to eat breakfast after your morning cardio; the portion size is larger than other meals that day because it not only replenishes the carbohydrate that was used during training and depleted during sleep but also restores the protein balance to support muscle growth. Meals will occasionally be skipped (this is unavoidable for most individuals with busy schedules). Make sure that one of these is not breakfast.

Drink tea and coffee devoid of sugar and cream.

It is advisable to avoid all the extra calories added to sugar and cream supply when drinking tea or coffee, though a modest amount of milk shouldn't hurt. It's amazing how many individuals eat perfectly healthy diets but still add eight to ten teaspoons of sugar to their daily coffee breaks to make up for the lack of simple sugars. The worst kind of nutrient can be included in an additional 160 calories per day by doing this.

Chew your food well.

The act of eating itself is a frequently disregarded element when it comes to good digestion and nutrient absorption. When food is properly chewed, saliva is added, and the meal is mashed up into an easily digestible state. The digestive process might not go as it should if food is not chewed thoroughly, and your body might not obtain the nutrients it needs.

Important Advice For Optimal Fat Loss & Muscle Growth

To guarantee proper energy levels before training, eat a healthy lunch one to two hours beforehand. Any type of vegetable, two pieces of fruit, low-fat cottage cheese with carrots, oatmeal with whey protein, or whole-meal sandwiches with chicken or beef can be had during this period. Eat roughly 30 minutes after exercising to refuel your energy. Take all six of the recommended daily meals. A persistent fat-burning effect (the after-burn) and enough energy levels for training will be made possible by doing this.

As stated in this plan, try to limit your intake of fatty foods and carbohydrates (rice, potatoes, veggies, and fruit) after 6 o'clock in the evening.
Consistency is the key to following this diet plan successfully. Every day's meals are based on the same food groups, with the exception of training days, when more protein and carbs are added after exercise and more calories are consumed overall. The diet choices are varied for diversity, but the same foods will be consumed every day because they serve your objectives the best.

The following formula can be used to calculate the precise amounts of each nutrient in each meal as well as the total for each meal: P=protein, C=carbohydrates, and F=fats. All dietary data is expressed in grams.

Chicken, potato, and rice cooking. I advise cooking a pot of skinless chicken breasts to be consumed over the course of two days (about four breasts). Rice and potatoes can both be boiled or baked and kept in Tupperware containers for up to three days. Everything here is done to save time.

Weekly Food List

Six 180-gram cans of tuna in water.

Eleven big chicken breasts in total.

Two sirloin steaks, one huge and two medium-sized.

Oatmeal, one package.

Rice weighing two kilograms.

Two wholemeal loaves of bread.

A single apple bag.

Sixty-two eggs.

A single potato sack.

No (or low) fat cottage cheese in five 250-gram containers.

Fresh fish weighing 1.5 to 2 pounds.

Two broccoli bags.

To be purchased as needed: whey protein, cod liver oil, and olive oil.

Chapter 9:

Techniques for consistently getting the finest outcomes.

How to Effortlessly Gain Muscle
A fundamental resistance training program is essential for effective muscular growth. The best approach to building muscle is to lift weights, according to Victoria Sekely, a doctor of physical therapy, certified strength and conditioning specialist, and run coach. Period."

According to the National Strength and Conditioning Association (NSCA), mechanical tension, muscle injury, and metabolic reaction are the three main components that cause hypertrophy. To harm the tissue, the tissue must first be overworked by increasing the load or resistance. A metabolic response begins as a result of the release of growth factors, which is triggered by the overload, which also causes an inflammatory reaction.

The NSCA advises determining your one-repetition maximum (1RM), or the most weight you can perform correctly and safely one time, to put this idea into reality. Try estimating your 1RM by first determining the weight you can lift for three to five repetitions, then estimating what your 1RM would be to prevent lifting weights that are too heavy. Generally speaking, if you can comfortably perform three sets of 10 repetitions at a specific resistance, you should increase the resistance and lower the number of reps. Hypertrophy is not induced by comfortable weightlifting without increasing the load.

To progressively increase strength if you are new to strength training, perform two to three rounds of six to twelve repetitions at 65% to 85% of your entire 1RM amount, resting for 60 seconds in between sets.

Try to complete two to three sets of six to twelve repetitions with 7.5 pounds, which is 75% of your total 1RM weight, for instance, if your 1RM is 10 pounds. If you are lifting a quantity that is closer to your complete 1RM weight, perform fewer reps. In both men and women, this process causes the highest levels of growth hormone and testosterone to be released, which helps in muscular growth.

This NSCA chart can assist you in estimating how much weight to use for your repetitions at 65% to 85% of your 1RM once you've determined how much weight you can safely use for 1RM. If you're just getting started, try to include this kind of strength training in your program two or three times per week; Depending on your level of experience, up to six times each week.

The 1RM you have is a moving target. You should be able to handle more weight as you gain muscle, so check your weight tolerance every few exercises and change your resistance as necessary. To put it another way, if in your first week of training your 1RM for a squat was 50 pounds, you'll need to reevaluate your development after a few exercises with this weight. In the third week of training, if your body can support greater weight, your 1RM can rise to 75 pounds. If your workouts are effective, your 1RM should gradually increase over time.

Start with bodyweight exercises, such as push-ups or squats without resistance, if you're new to fitness and strength training, advises Sekely, before adding weight. She goes on to say, "Before adding a heavy load, it's important to feel comfortable with the mechanics of a movement pattern." Prepared to begin developing muscle? Take into account this professional advice.

1. Be Particular

Focus your workout on a specific muscle or set of muscles if you want to gain muscle. You can lift more weight by including multi-joint workouts that involve the target muscle, according to Sekely. For instance, if you want to bulk up your biceps, practice performing exercises like bicep curls that directly load that muscle. It may also be advantageous to perform a multi-joint exercise that targets your biceps and engages larger muscle groups, like as a dumbbell row, which works the latissimus dorsi, or lats, as well as other shoulder muscles.

Before beginning your muscle-building adventure, Sekely advises speaking with a strength coach or physical therapist for advice on the ideal exercises for you to complete in order to achieve your objectives, especially if you have a history of injuries or are new to strength training.

2. Consume protein

It's essential to give your muscles the right nutrition if you want to increase muscle healthily and effectively. When cells try to rebuild muscle fibers, which must be accompanied by a sufficient protein intake from diet, muscle hypertrophy results. If you don't give your body enough protein, it won't be able to rebuild those muscle fibers, according to Sekely.

"Protein is the most important and essential component of nutrition and the foundation of muscle gain," notwithstanding the importance of carbohydrate intake. Dr. Graham advises consuming 1 gram of protein for every pound of body weight if you're wondering how much protein you need to gain muscle. Chicken, eggs, salmon, Greek yogurt, lean beef, and soybeans are all excellent sources of protein. And while you're concentrating on eating, make sure you drink enough water to stay adequately hydrated.

3. Sleep

Anyone trying to gain muscle should make sure they get adequate sleep. According to, our cells must enter a phase of repair and regeneration for 7 to 8 hours each night. Lack of sleep makes the process of healing injured tissue less effective, which can result in subpar results and even injury. A high-protein diet and plenty of sleep are both important for maximizing the effects of hypertrophy.

4. Don't Give Up

Keep in mind that your statistics should be changing as you train. Your 1RM and training program must expand along with you if you're actually gaining muscle and strength. For ongoing growth, regular strength evaluations and a well-thought-out exercise progression are essential. If you continue to lift the same amount of weight, you won't initiate the process of muscle damage and regeneration necessary to develop larger muscles. However, if you lift too much, you risk doing more harm than good and getting hurt.

5. Inhale

Working on your legs, arms, or core while controlling your breathing will help your muscles and heart get the oxygen they require to safely complete the challenging workouts without raising your blood pressure.

Abdominal bracing can assist protect your body from harm by providing a more stable base from which to lift. Start by inhaling to do this kind of breathing. Create a strong trunk and foundation for lifting by gently drawing your gut in as you exhale, as if you were getting ready to take a punch to the stomach. On your exhale, start lifting big objects.